D0097019

The RACE IS RUN

One Step at a Time

Every Woman's Guide to Taking Charge of BREAST CANCER & My Personal Story

by

NANCY G. BRINKER
Founder of the Susan G. Komen Breast Cancer Foundation and Race for the Cure©

with

CATHERINE McEVILY HARRIS

THE SUMMIT PUBLISHING GROUP • ARLINGTON, TEXAS

THE SUMMIT PUBLISHING GROUP

One Arlington Centre
1112 E. Copeland Road, Fifth Floor
Arlington, Texas 76011

95 96 97 98 99   5 4 3 2 1

LIBRARY OF CONGRESS CATALOGING-IN PUBLICATION DATA
Brinker, Nancy.
The race is run one step at a time: every woman's guide to taking charge of breast cancer / Nancy Brinker with Catherine McEvily Harris ; witha foreword by Samuel Broder. — Newly rev.
p. cm.
Previously published : New York : Simon & Schuster. 1991.
Includes bibliographical references and index.
ISBN 1-56530-182-X
1. Breast — Cancer — Popular works. I. Harris, Catherine McEvily. II. Title.
RC280.B8B73 1995
362.1'9699449 — dc20   95–24204
                                                                CIP

Cover and book design by David Sims

DISCARD

THE RACE IS RUN ONE STEP AT A TIME

Presented by:

The Arkansas Chapter of the
Susan G. Komen Breast Cancer Foundation

Phone 1-800-I M AWARE

To my sister, Susan G. Komen;

To our dear mother, Eleanor Newman Goodman,
and our father, Marvin Goodman, for creating her;

To my husband and son, for helping me keep her memory alive;

And to the Susan G. Komen Breast Cancer Foundation,
through which her spirit will live forever.

Contents

Acknowledgments

I find it difficult to thank everyone who has helped me with this book, as the list would include all of my family, mentors, volunteers, and the staff of the Komen Foundation, and, of course, the many courageous breast cancer survivors and patients. But, in addition to these many wonderful people who helped me with the first edition of this book, I would like to thank those whose time and effort went into updating the important medical information contained in this edition.

To Dr. Fritz Barton, Dr. Phil Evans, Dr. John Minna, Dr. George Peters, Dr. R. Pickett Scruggs and Dr. Victor Vogel for their medical advice and wise counsel, and to Linda Frame, RN, MS, OCN for her time and effort.

To Midge Moseley who worked so diligently on the editing and rewriting of this book. I am hopeful that it will become even more useful and continue to educate and comfort breast cancer patients, families, survivors and anyone who is confronted with this disease. It has strengthened my commitment to all patients, families, physicians, nurses, donors, and all those whose lives are touched by breast cancer, especially the 1.5 million who will be diagnosed this decade.

And my special thanks to the wonderful staff and volunteers of the Susan G. Komen Breast Cancer Foundation, who carry on tirelessly in the fight against breast cancer.

℮

Foreword

by

DR. SAMUEL BRODER

Former Director, National Cancer Institute

This year approximately one hundred eighty thousand women will be diagnosed as having breast cancer; approximately forty-six thousand will die. The search for a cure has been a difficult road. We live in an era of rapid technological changes, and there have been many advances in basic science and clinical practice. But there is still much to learn. Breast cancer patients with a practical knowledge of the disease have a great advantage.

The Race Is Run One Step at a Time will make the road considerably easier—at least easy enough to follow. Scientists and physicians often forget they are speaking to people unacquainted with cancer terminology. This book makes the medical jargon clear and meaningful.

Nancy Brinker's book is not intended for women alone, but for everyone. Breast cancer touches the lives of all of us. This important volume gives women, and the men and children who love and care about them, a starting point—a compass with which they can begin their race to obtain information. In telling her personal story, Brinker teaches by example, and, in outlining her knowledge, she provides a model for the informed patient.

Bench science will never be adequately transferred to the

clinic without a population of informed patients. An educated population is the best ally of physicians dedicated to preventing, diagnosing, and treating breast cancer.

Nancy Brinker is driven to do something about this disease. She founded the Komen Foundation—an organization that supports research and training, and is making a real difference—to honor a sister who died of breast cancer. During the course of Brinker's crusade, the disease eventually threatened her own life. With the establishment of the Komen Foundation she turned her personal battle with cancer into a public mission. With the publication of this book, Nancy Brinker is making yet another important contribution.

Breast cancer is an exceedingly high priority of the National Cancer Institute. Through research, we have learned how certain hormones or growth factors can lead to abnormal growth patterns, ultimately contributing to the development of cancer. We now know about special genes (oncogenes) that might directly contribute to cancer. A newer class of genes (suppressor genes) can prevent the malignant state to begin with. Two genes (BRCA-1 and BRCA-2) have been identified as the cause of certain types of familial breast cancer. As we proceed, this kind of research will make a tremendous difference in locating a cure, but there is also much we can do now to battle the disease. Regular mammogram and clinical exams can have great success in detecting and curing breast cancer. New approaches to surgery and follow-up chemotherapy or hormonal therapy can make a big difference in a woman's survival and in the quality of her life. Multidisciplinary cooperation can make breast cancer treatment a team effort. Better information services, such as the Physicians Data Query (PDQ) system can provide up-to-the-minute information for physicians and surgeons. And information services for the general public can be enormously effective.

The first step, however, begins with the patient and her family. That's what real cancer information is all about.

Introduction

The last thing in the world I ever thought I'd do was write a book. The truth is, I never thought I could sit still long enough to complete one. I would never have imagined myself having so much to say on any one particular subject.

Nothing in life is to be feared. It is only to be understood.

MADAME CURIE

Of course, I never imagined I'd be living my life without the company of my sister, Susan Goodman Komen. Growing up in Peoria, Illinois, Suzy and I were filled with childhood dreams. Our dreams were always very different, but that didn't seem to matter because we also had many things in common. We spent endless hours discussing in intricate detail the paths our lives were likely to take. Suzy's always pertained to having a handsome husband, a family, and a home in Peoria, while mine took on a much grander vision. I wanted all of the above and more. I can remember as far back as when I was three years old plotting and scheming ways to get *out* of Peoria. I wanted more excitement and stimulation than any hometown could offer.

Even as a little girl I always had high aspirations. Leading a quiet, sedentary life was not an option—I had to see the world. I had no way of knowing what a cataclysmic series of events would have to take place before that vision would become reality.

Regardless of how our lives were to differ, Suzy and I always planned to take care of our parents together when the time came, share a room in the "old folks' home" one day, and compare stories about our husbands, kids, and grandchildren. It never dawned on me that things could turn out so differently. No, I must admit that not one of our many childhood dreams included breast cancer. Even I, with the most vivid of imaginations, never thought about what it would be like to spend three years watching this disease slowly and painfully suck the life out of my best friend. Not once did I fantasize about what it would be like to hear those dreaded words, "It's cancer," referring to my own breast. Nor did I think for a minute that I'd start a national foundation for breast cancer research in my sister's memory.

As all too often happens in the game of life, I was dealt an unexpected hand of cards. God knows, I'm not the first woman to experience such a hand. I'm not even the first woman to put her story on paper. There have been others before me who have bravely told their stories to the world and were far more prolific than I.

So, why am I doing this? What would make a person share such painful and intimate details of her life? Allow me to offer a statistic that says it all:

During the ten years of the Vietnam War,
fifty-eight thousand men and women died.
During that same ten-year period,
three hundred thirty thousand women died of breast cancer.

Breast cancer is our country's number-two killer of women.

Thirty years ago a woman had a one-in-fourteen chance of developing breast cancer in her lifetime. Today that figure has grown to one in nine. It is a disease that strikes women in the prime of their most productive years of life, often attacking its victims between the ages of thirty and fifty. It is also a disease that tears into the depths of a woman's soul and threatens what she often cherishes most, her femininity and her self-image. Today, a woman over thirty-five is at the forefront of an exciting era. She's at a new pinnacle in terms of career, family, romance, and sexuality. Often she is starting over in one or more of these areas. Breast cancer threatens to take it all away. And what it leaves in its place is a woman with a disease that is hard to discuss, difficult to endure, and nearly impossible to prevent.

Fifty years ago, when a person was diagnosed with breast cancer it meant the worst. Gloom and doom hovered over that person like a dark rain cloud. And, whether it was mentioned aloud or not, a slow and painful death was almost always envisioned by all. Fortunately, times have changed. No one has to give in to breast cancer anymore or assume that it will eventually be the victor. Nor should one assume that engaging in battle with breast cancer will permanently devalue her quality of life. I have personally witnessed the best and worst of the situation. My sister died a slow and painful death. She was not educated about the disease and neither were the people on whom she relied most. Because of Suzy's death and my promise to her on her deathbed, I have made it a point to learn everything I can about breast cancer. I'm still learning every day.

When cancer was discovered in my own breast, of course I was frightened. I cried and experienced all of the reactions you would expect of a woman diagnosed with a life-threatening disease. But I had an advantage Suzy didn't have—an advantage you'll have, too: I had a pretty good idea what my options were and knew where to go for the answers I was missing. I assembled what I affectionately refer to as my "A Team" of experts and together we met the disease head on. The point I want to make is this: After having my breast removed, receiving high doses of chemotherapy, and undergoing reconstructive surgery, my life is fuller and more active than ever before. It has not deteriorated one bit. I work out nearly every day, am active at The Susan G. Komen Breast Cancer Foundation (which I founded after Suzy's death), and pursue other business interests—none of which is as strenuous as keeping up with my son. The two major differences in my life now compared to before I had cancer are that today I am much busier and I appreciate the value of good health as never before. I am telling you this because I want you to know what I know. Even if you find yourself diagnosed with breast cancer, it does not have to mean the end of the world. Dealing with this disease requires a plan of action. A good football team maps out its winning strategy. So should you. But before you can do that, you must know something about the game.

So far, there is no cure. But there *is* hope. When breast cancer is detected in its earliest stages, there is a greater-than-90-percent, five-year survival rate. My cancer was detected early; my sister's was not. I had the opportunity to marshal my possibilities; my sister did not. I am living a full and happy life with a son and a husband who are more precious to me than anything in the world. My sister left behind two young children, a very lonely husband, two heartbroken parents, many wonderful friends, and me.

My object is not to frighten you with statistics on breast cancer—quite the contrary. Suzy was frightened, so frightened that her fear paralyzed her judgment. She is dead. This is not to say my sister's death could have been prevented. Ten percent of all breast cancers are so aggressive and grow so fast they simply *outsmart* all forms of treatment, and that very well might have been the case with Suzy's. But I believe in my heart that had all of us been better informed about the facts, had we known enough to try all the options available, her life might have been prolonged, if not saved. Those precious few years would have provided her two children with more of the nurturing they so desperately needed. The prospect of discovering cancer in yourself or someone you love is one of the most terrifying feelings imaginable. But believe me when I tell you that you are better off if you feel anger along with the terror. Cancer is one of those enemies that needs to be dealt with immediately. Anger, focused positively, provides you with strength.

The purpose of writing this book is to empower you by helping you to deal with the considerable amount of information you *need* to know in order to stand a fighting chance against breast cancer. I have learned a great deal over the years. God knows, the opportunity has presented itself. My sister's life was taken by breast cancer, and my own life was threatened by the same disease. Now breast cancer is my career. The knowledge I've accumulated wasn't part of my plan. It was born from the necessity of dealing with the hand of cards I was dealt. Unfortunately, I couldn't throw my hand in—you can't either. I don't believe, however, that the only way to learn important lessons in life is by making your own mistakes.

The most powerful gift of the written word is its ability to reach out and teach those who may follow an already traveled path. Learn from my mistakes and the mistakes of my family. Learn from our triumphs, too. I wasn't born with any phenomenal gifts. I am just a regular woman who grew up in midwestern America. I do not presume to pose as a medical authority. But what I have found in my quest for knowledge is that the dark, mysterious picture which is automatically conjured up in many minds by the word *science* is not that dark and not that mysterious. It is a matter of deciphering the code, as it were, and learning the language. Once I understood what all those pathologists, radiologists, oncologists, and surgeons were talking about, I was able to think more clearly and make intelligent decisions about my own cancer.

I have structured the book into two parts. In Part One, I will tell you what happened to Suzy and me. The story might be, at times, painful to read; I know it was painful to write. We were two sisters with the same disease. One of us lived; one of us died. We each handled our breast cancer very differently, both medically and mentally. In those differences lies the theme of this book. I fought my illness with everything I had. My sister didn't have my knowledge or experience. She couldn't have fought the same way I did.

Part Two is directed at you, the reader. I will take you through what is thought to be the basics. There is a lot to know about the breasts, not just about breast cancer but about benign breast disease and how the breasts function normally. If you have a true sense of how your body works without a problem, you will then develop a sort of *sixth sense* which will make you acutely aware should anything out of the ordinary occur. As we delve into the specifics of the disease itself, I will try to give you the information you'll need most in order to combat breast cancer. The truth, as I know it, is that the only way to overcome an obstacle in life is to follow a well-charted plan. We'll talk about treatment, old and new, both surgical and nonsurgical. Things are changing every day in the world of medicine. We'll also talk about what's on the horizon in terms of forthcoming research and what is being done to help overcome the emotional aspect of this very personal and intimate disease. And, finally, we'll talk about what little is known about the causes of breast cancer and the preventive measures assumed at this time.

Until a cure is found, we must fight with the only weapon we have—knowledge. No, I am not a doctor, but I can assist you in finding one. I would like to help you put together your own "A Team" of experts. And on this team, it will be up to you to call the shots. We all have to take responsibility for our own bodies. We can solicit the help of the finest experts in the country, but the final choices have to be our own. We can't make wise choices without valid information. For far too long the majority of information has been left in the hands of men. Breast cancer is largely a woman's disease (slightly more than one-half of 1 percent of all diagnosed cases of breast cancer are found in men), yet it is mostly men on whom we depend for research and treatment. I often wonder just how much closer we'd be to finding a cure if the statistics were as high on breast cancer cases diagnosed in men as they are in women. If I am successful in my purpose for writing this book, by the time you finish the last page you will have more knowledge and feel better armed against this formidable opponent. Ultimately, you will have the ability to make informed decisions about your own health and well-being.

Through the Susan G. Komen Breast Cancer Foundation I have been able to keep my sister's memory alive. The women and men who have become cherished members of our cause have helped, each in his or her own way, to fill the vast void in my heart left by her death. Suzy didn't want anyone to suffer the way she did. I don't either. The good news is...you might not have to.

About Nancy Brinker

When Nancy's sister Susan died of breast cancer at the age of thirty-six, Nancy promised herself she would fulfill Suzy's plea to help others confronted with the disease. In 1982, she founded the Dallas-based Susan G. Komen Breast Cancer Foundation, which today is a leader in the field of breast cancer research funding, education, and legislative advocacy. Since its inception the foundation has raised more than $39 million, funded more than two hundred national grants, and is the nation's largest private funder of research dedicated solely to breast cancer.

Nancy created the foundation's trademark Race for the Cure® series of five-kilometer runs, which is the nation's largest women's race series and has helped the foundation raise funds for screening and education projects in local communities across the country and for the foundation's research grant program.

In 1986, President Ronald Reagan appointed Nancy as one of only six laypersons to the prestigious National Cancer Advisory Board. In 1991, President George Bush appointed Nancy to the three-member President's Cancer Panel, where in 1992 she chaired the Subcommittee on Breast Cancer.

Continually looking for new ways to reach out to the American public, educate consumers, and change behavior, Nancy created her own for-profit company, In Your Corner, Inc.,™ in 1994 to provide the retail marketplace with educational, reliable, and entertaining health and wellness information.

She currently serves on the corporate board of directors of Caremark International and Physician's Reliance Network, Inc., as well as on several nonprofit boards including Harvard University School of Public Health and University of Texas M. D. Anderson Cancer Center.

Herself a breast cancer survivor, Nancy has testified before Congress on major breast cancer and health-care issues and has appeared on most every major television news program. She has received numerous awards for her work in the field of breast cancer, including:

- Dallas County Medical Society Award of the Year
- Vincent T. Lombardi Cancer Center Symbol of Caring Award
- Marie Lombardi Humanitarian Award
- Layman's Award of the Society of Surgical Oncology
- Fox Chase Cancer Center Reimann Honor Award
- Hadassah Myrtle Wreath Award
- University of Illinois Distinguished Alumni Award and Alumni Achievement Award
- American Society of Clinical Oncology (ASCO) Award
- Albert Einstein College of Medicine Lizette H. Sarnoff Award for Volunteer Services
- Voted into Texas Women's Hall of Fame
- Texas Governor's Award for Outstanding National Service
- Association of Community Cancer Centers Annual Award
- National Association of Women's Health Professionals Special Services Award

- Woman of Distinction Award from Birmingham-Southern College
- Gib Lewis Award for Excellence in Cancer Control

A "distinguished" graduate of the University of Illinois, Nancy and her husband, restaurant industry leader Norman E. Brinker, and son, Eric, reside in Dallas, Texas. She has a terrific extended family including stepchildren and their families, her parents, cousins, and her late sister Suzy's husband, Stan, and their children, Stephanie and Scott.

PART ONE

My Sister
and I

CHAPTER ONE

Suzy's Story

The first time I can remember hearing the words *breast cancer* was back in 1956. I was ten years old and living in Peoria, Illinois, with my parents, Eleanor and Marvin Goodman, and my older sister, Susan. Our home was on a quiet, tree-lined street in a peaceful neighborhood where every neighbor was a friend, much like a scene right out of *Father Knows Best*. It was a traditional life and the rules were clearly laid out. Dinner was served on a white tablecloth and good manners were mandatory. Mealtime was family time in the Goodman household and that meant no interruptions. No boyfriends, no phone calls—no nothing. Dad was the family leader and authoritarian, of that there was no doubt. Although we always felt loved, he was a very strict man who demanded respect. It was this discipline that gave us our structure and me my drive. It would hurt his feelings terribly if I said I thought he loved Suzy more, but their relationship *was* different. Suzy was his first child and born a bit premature. She was a meeker and milder child, not to mention a lot smaller than me. He idolized little Suzy and in his eyes she could

> *It is better to light one candle than curse the darkness.*
>
> MOTTO OF THE CHRISTOPHER SOCIETY

do no wrong. The truth of the matter is, she *did* no wrong. I, on the other hand, started out on the wrong foot from the beginning. I was supposed to be a boy. I weighed in at over a hundred pounds in second grade and had all the grace and poise of a baby elephant. I wasn't nearly as cuddly as my sister, but I had a quick, curious mind. Dad simply expected more from me. Looking back now, I'm grateful for being taught to push harder, but back then it was sometimes hard to swallow.

My mother has always been a woman of amazing patience, kindness, and inner strength. She allowed my father to "run" the family, yet she was the one who knew all our secrets, kept all our confidences. When something needed to be done, we depended on her for results. And she never let us down. Mom was a great mediator between my father and everyone else. She was and still is the world's best peacekeeper. She ran the Girl Scouts in Peoria, was a tireless charity volunteer, never missed a PTA meeting, was usually in the kitchen baking cookies when Suzy and I came home from school, and always had dinner waiting for my father at the end of each day. And she did it all with a smile on her face. But my mother's finest gift to the world is her ability to find the humor in any situation.

Suzy and I were unable to suppress squeals of joy when we were informed one night at dinner that we were going to visit our favorite aunt, Rose, all the way in New York City. Since Suzy was thirteen, Mom and Dad felt we were old enough to make the trip by plane to the big city by ourselves. To me, it was to be an exciting adventure, never mind the fact that our parents would put us safely on the plane and Aunt Rose would be waiting at the other end to pick us up.

Anyway, that night after dinner my mother came into our bedroom while we were dutifully doing our homework and told us she had something to talk to us about. She wanted to remind us that although Aunt Rose was feeling great and looked good she had been very sick with breast cancer and had had an operation called a mastectomy. Suzy quickly jumped in and told Mom we both knew about the operation and she didn't need to explain the details of Aunt Rose's surgery. In the back of my mind I had an idea what a mastectomy was, but I could tell, even then, that the subject was uncomfortable for Suzy—so I didn't ask any questions. Any subject with even so much as a hint of violence, pain, or mutilation would upset her terribly. I remember when Suzy's stallion was being gelded, she ran away screaming with her hands over her face while I sat up in a nearby tree and, although I winced and covered my eyes, through parted fingers I watched the whole thing with great interest.

By the time we saw Aunt Rose, so ebullient and full of life, laughing and flirting with her new husband (her fourth), all thoughts that she had once been sick passed completely from our minds. We listened intently while Rose told of her exotic safari in Africa. Oh, how I admired this woman. She did anything she wanted to do, any time she wanted to do it. She was independent and free-spirited and I wanted to be just like her. Suzy admired her too, but for different reasons. She saw in Aunt Rose the epitome of femininity. And she was right. Aunt Rose was truly glamorous. She entered and exited every room just like Loretta Young, with a chiffon scarf floating through the air. Her clothes were always beautiful and her perfume wafted behind her in a way that left her on your mind long after she had gone. And she did have a way with men! She knew how to get men to do anything and everything she wanted them to do, and she did it by making those men feel as if they were the most important and wonderful thing in her life.

On our third night in New York, something happened that would have a lasting effect on Suzy and me. Aunt Rose had taken us shopping, skating, and to the theater. We had had a long day and Suzy and I were simply exhausted. As sometimes happens when two sisters are both tired, Suzy and I got into a little squabble before bedtime. Whatever the argument was about we just couldn't seem to resolve it between ourselves this time, so Suzy marched in to discuss the matter with Aunt Rose. All of a sudden Suzy came tearing back into our room in a hysterical frenzy. I had never seen her so upset. She looked terrified. When I finally got her to calm down long enough to tell me what was wrong, she reported that she had gone into Aunt Rose's room without knocking and had accidentally seen the scars on her chest. She said they were terribly gruesome and she couldn't understand how Aunt Rose had lived through such mutilation. Naturally, I had to check out the situation for myself. So I tiptoed back to Aunt Rose's room and quietly opened the door to get a quick peek. Well, Suzy wasn't kidding. Not only were the scars severe, but her chest looked concave and burned from high-voltage cobalt treatments. I could even faintly see her heart beating through thin, purple skin. Aunt Rose had had what is known as a Halsted radical mastectomy on her left side. Although the procedure is rarely done today, it was considered common treatment for breast cancer for nearly a hundred years and was certainly common back then in 1956. The Halsted radical removes not only the breast but all the underarm lymph nodes, the chest muscles, and some additional fat and skin. The truth is, her particular operation *was* unattractive. I have since learned more about the procedure and realize that hers was poorly done. But, as I softly closed the door and began to walk back to Suzy I heard Aunt Rose singing happily to her husband. I decided Aunt Rose didn't need my sympathy. Aunt Rose was living a fuller, richer, more exciting life than anyone else I knew. If her mastectomy didn't bother her, why should it bother me? But Suzy never got over it. The memory of Aunt Rose's chest haunted her forever.

As we got older, Suzy and I became just about as close as two sisters can get. Suzy was the perfect older sister. She was beautiful and kind and loving, not only to me but to everyone. There was a goodness and gentleness about my sister that went unnoticed by no one. She was the star of our hometown of Peoria, the high school homecoming queen, the college beauty queen. She was everyone's darling and I don't think there was a soul who ever met her who didn't fall in love with her—men, women, and children alike. I worshipped Suzy and used to follow her around everywhere. She never seemed to mind. If she did, she never showed it. I, on the other hand, was bigger, heavier, and taller than most of my friends *and* her friends. I developed my own way of getting attention. I was a tomboy and a mischief-maker and delighted in nothing more than spending hours galloping around on horseback. Suzy tried desperately to teach me about all the pretty things in life: how to fix my hair, apply makeup, and coordinate my wardrobe. None of it seemed to work. I was still a big, sort of clumsy girl with two left feet. The boys didn't know I was alive, except that I was Susan Goodman's younger, "bookish" sister. The only frustration we ever had with each other was that it bothered me that Suzy seemed content to stay right where she was just as it bothered her to constantly see the discontent in my eyes.

Suzy came back to Peoria when she graduated from college and got a job modeling locally. Eventually, she married her college sweetheart, Stan Komen. Stan and Suzy had a very good marriage. Although they were unable to have children of their own, they soon adopted two beautiful babies, Scott and Stephanie. Suzy had everything she wanted: a loving husband and a family of her own.

College, for me, was the first time I felt I belonged anywhere. At the University of Illinois, the baby fat came off as did the braces. I was active in many school projects and finally began to have confidence in myself. I felt independent and responsible and ready to take on the world. After graduating, I packed up my

Suzy, Dad (Marvin Goodman), and me, 1952

With Suzy and Mother (Ellie Goodman), and Aunt Rose and her husband, whom she married after her radical mastectomy.

bags and moved to Dallas, home of my father's older sister, Aunt Ruth. As a child, I had spent many vacations in Texas and often dreamed of one day living amid the wide open ranchland. When Dad finally agreed to the move, or at least realized he couldn't stop me, he made it clear that I would have to support myself.

So I walked into Neiman Marcus and told the personnel director my situation. "Look," I said, "my parents are not happy about my being in Texas. I need a job, and I need a good one." I started as an executive trainee and worked up to an assistant couture buyer. It was at Neiman Marcus that I met my first husband. The marriage, by all counts, was a mistake, except for one wonderful miracle—my son, Eric.

Although we were separated by distance, Suzy and I spoke every day by phone in the late afternoon. Our daily conversations were something I grew to depend on and cherish. She kept me up-to-date on what was happening in Peoria and I filled her in on my life in Dallas. We discussed our children, our husbands, and our careers at great length. Suzy's calm, kind-hearted way was a perfect contrast to my frantic, impatient nature. In a way, I was her third child and she was my second mother. Above all, we made each other laugh.

It was about this time that Suzy and I became aware we both had a common and nonthreatening condition called fibrocystic disease. This is a lumpiness in the breast caused by the breast's response to hormonal levels as they change from month to month. Lumpy, or cystic, breasts are often accompanied by pain or tenderness that fluctuates with the menstrual cycle, becoming more noticeable and painful just before your period begins. Fibrocystic disease is by far the most frequently occurring breast disorder and nearly all women's breasts develop some degree of this condition at one time or another. We will talk about fibrocystic disease in more detail in chapter 3, but the point I want to make now is that neither Suzy nor I was concerned in the least about our condition. Occasionally, Suzy's doctor would perform what is called a needle aspiration. Using a needle and syringe to withdraw fluid or a small amount of tissue from a breast lump can show whether that lump is a fluid-filled cyst or a solid mass. Hers were fluid-filled cysts and by puncturing the lump with a needle, the mass drained and disappeared. Regardless of how it sounds, this procedure was, again, nothing that caused her alarm. Our doctors assured us that eight out of ten lumps were not dangerous in any way and that we had nothing to worry about. Besides, we both felt young and invincible.

As if it were yesterday, I can remember the phone call I received from Suzy one Tuesday afternoon. Her doctor had found a lump that was not a cyst. He recommended a biopsy. A biopsy is the surgical removal and microscopic examination of tissue to see if cancer cells are present. Now, you must understand that my sister was the most nurturing, loving woman in the world. She took it upon herself to help everyone who crossed her path. And, by force of habit, we not only allowed her to comfort us when we needed it, we grew to depend on it. Hearing uneasiness in her voice, as much as she tried to hide it, was unnatural. And it frightened me. Of course, my parents and I tried to make light of the situation and tell Suzy we were sure that everything would be fine. But, to be honest, we weren't sure at all. Not at all. And although none of us mentioned it, the memory of Aunt Rose had been brought back to life vividly in all our minds.

I decided to fly home to Peoria. Suzy said it wasn't necessary, that she would call me when they found out the results. I insisted on coming anyway, saying that I wanted to be there for the celebration when the tests came back negative. But when I got off the plane, my father was waiting there alone with an expression on his face I will never forget. He didn't have to say a word. *At the age of thirty-three, Suzy had breast cancer.*

What happened from this point on is still difficult for me to

Me (right) with my best friend, Suzy, 1975.

talk about because I am so much more knowledgeable on the subject today. *If I had only known then what I know now.*

The truth of the matter is that growing up in the small town of Peoria, our family had been treated our whole lives by one doctor. He was a nice man and a fine physician, and we relied on him for all of our childhood illnesses. He was probably the last of the kind, an older doctor who still made house calls and was a friend not only to us, but to everyone he treated. Suzy trusted him with her cancer the same way she trusted him with her measles. *Mistake number one.* None of us knew enough to inquire about seeking information from a major cancer center near our town or from a group of physicians associated with one in Peoria. He was our doctor. Period.

The most difficult concept to grasp about cancer, I think, is the fact that when it is first detected the patient usually feels just fine. There is rarely any pain associated with breast cancer in its early stages. So when you are told you've got a life-threatening disease, and the treatment sounds more heinous than the thought of a little lump in the breast, it is understandable that a woman uneducated about cancer might opt for no treatment at all. Such was the case with Suzy. My sister was terrified, naturally, but adamant against having a mastectomy. She wasn't vain in a negative sense; she was just extremely feminine and enjoyed every part of being a woman. That included having breasts. Two of them.

Our family doctor called in a surgeon to review Suzy's case. It is important, if you are to learn from our mistakes, that I tell you a little bit about this surgeon. He was very handsome, very suave, and seemed very self-confident. He told us that her cancer was a medullary carcinoma and there were no lymph nodes involved. I will go into more detail about this medical terminology later on, but briefly what I understood him to mean was that in his opinion her cancer had not spread or metastasized to other parts of her body. According to Suzy, this surgeon—I will refer to him as Dr. Smith (not his real name)—told Suzy he could cure her. Even the most respected cancer experts in the country (which Dr. Smith was certainly not) talk about recovery in terms of surviving cancer or remission. They refrain from using the word *cure* because cancer can recur.

But that, of course, is exactly what Suzy wanted to hear, and who could blame her? Like many women, and for that matter men, too, Suzy was of the frame of mind that the doctor was always right. She believed in Dr. Smith without question, and when he smiled at her and said everything would be fine, she willingly gave herself up to this man. Suzy really didn't want to know everything there was to know about the disease, she just wanted him to make her better. She wanted not to be frightened anymore, she wanted to look normal, and she wanted to go back to being a healthy wife and mother to her children.

Dr. Smith suggested performing a subcutaneous mastectomy, a procedure in which the outside of the breast is left intact but an incision is made and the breast tissue is removed. He would then do an implant ten days later. She would be left with a small scar but no more cancer. Suzy felt it was her best option. She was not referred to an oncologist—a cancer specialist—for a second opinion. The year was 1977 and although cancer treatments weren't nearly as sophisticated as they are today, we wish she had been offered the chance to participate in a clinical trial at a major comprehensive cancer center. A clinical trial is an experimental study conducted with cancer patients, usually to evaluate a new treatment. Each study is designed to answer specific scientific questions. A patient is randomly assigned to one of several treatments with the scientific goals being to measure the success of one over the other. At that time, they would sometimes compare a patient receiving a certain formula of drugs with a patient receiving no drugs at all. And because the assignments were random, there was always the chance she would have been put in a group without drugs, but at least she would have been part of a closely monitored study conducted by doctors at a comprehensive cancer center.

The rest of us tried very hard among ourselves to figure out what was best for her. But at that time, we were certainly no experts. Suzy was very upset and Stan wanted to keep her calm, so he went along with what she wanted. My mother instinctively had a lot of questions, but was afraid to push too hard, fearing Suzy might decide to do nothing rather than go for more intense treatment. My father was devastated and did not know where to turn or what to do. It was very sad. I, being the rebel, wanted Suzy to get out of Peoria and have a second opinion at a comprehensive cancer center. To me, both our family doctor and Dr. Smith, while their intentions were good, lacked the sophistication and exposure that can only be found through years of concentrated study in a given field. Their attention had been too diversified, treating everything from chicken pox to appendectomies. These are normal and admirable credentials in small-town physicians, but in my opinion, not good enough for my sister's condition at that time. I wanted Suzy to have the best, I wanted her to come to Texas. But she wanted to stay in Peoria where she was comfortable and loved. And that is exactly what she did.

After Suzy's surgery, my parents, Stan, and I were all at the hospital anxiously awaiting the results. Dr. Smith walked confidently in the room and said, "You can relax; we got it all. I believe she's cured." My heart sank because I knew enough to know that *cure* is a very difficult word to use in reference to cancer. If it is used at all, it is more likely to be spoken after a five-year period has passed without a recurrence.

Let me set the record straight about Suzy's doctors: Neither of them had anything but good intentions, nor did they want anything less than good health for her. Both of these doctors loved my sister and wanted nothing more than to see her well. And she loved them. Suzy felt that the better she knew her doctors, the closer the doctor/patient relationship, the better the prognosis. She felt that because these doctors were her *friends*, they wouldn't let her down. They *couldn't* let her down because friends don't do that to each other. Aside from radiation, I don't remember other treatment or adjuvant therapy being suggested. Nowadays it is common to perform additional tests such as bone scans, liver scans, or CAT scans to determine whether the cancer has metastasized.

For the next five months or so, Suzy felt pretty good. She was convinced she was cured. When I suggested she secure a second opinion just to be sure, she became very sensitive. After all, her doctor had told her she was fine. I was back in Dallas, having my own problems dealing with a failing marriage. Suzy didn't want to talk about her illness so, God bless her, she spent hours on the phone each day counseling me. I was concerned because Suzy had a shallow cough that wouldn't go away and she really didn't seem to have her energy back. She was cheerful and happy, but that old zing and sparkle just wasn't there. I didn't dare suggest that she was still sick. How could I, when Suzy was so optimistic? Quietly, I worried.

Before six months had gone by, our worst nightmare became a reality. Suzy found another lump. This time it was under her arm. Despite everyone's optimism her cancer had spread.

I wanted to take Suzy to the M. D. Anderson Cancer Center in Houston because through my contacts in Dallas, I had learned this facility was one of the most comprehensive cancer centers in the country. Suzy wasn't familiar with M. D. Anderson, but she knew about the Mayo Clinic so that's where she went next. It was at Mayo where we learned that her cancer had metastasized (spread) to her lung and under her arm. There was a tumor the size of a quarter in the upper part of her right lung and suspicious shadows elsewhere. Their recommendation was thirty days of radiation and then to "watch it." Well I, for one, was tired of "watching." I wanted to see some results.

Terror, rage, sadness, and above all, a feeling of complete and utter helplessness invaded me. Why was this happening to Suzy, of all people? What in the hell had she ever done to deserve to be so sick and so frightened? Although no one said anything aloud, we all knew my sister was now fighting for her life. *And it all happened so quickly.* She tried to keep up a brave front and would often talk of plans for the future.

A major turning point in Suzy's struggle for survival came from a surprising source, Mrs. Betty Ford. The year was 1978 and Mrs. Ford had finished a successful bout with breast cancer as First Lady. The whole country was shocked and saddened with the news of her breast cancer and mastectomy. Her bravery touched a place inside of Suzy that none of us could possibly understand because we hadn't gone through it ourselves. In Betty Ford, my sister found new strength. "Nan," she said, "if Mrs. Ford can admit she has breast cancer and tell the whole world she intends to fight it, well, then so can I." The doctors at Mayo suggested Suzy have radiation therapy, which is a treatment using high-energy rays to damage (burn) cancer cells and stop them from growing. She did have the radiation but it was not successful in slowing her disease. The cancer was out of control and there wasn't a damn thing we could do about it. But we had to try. Thank goodness, Suzy's plastic surgeon in Peoria suggested she try M. D. Anderson. I guess there is something about hearing advice from a nonfamily member that allows it to sink in. It didn't matter; I was thrilled she had decided to give Houston a try.

Through contacts I had made when helping with a charity benefit for M. D. Anderson I was able to get Suzy an appointment with an oncologist (a doctor who specializes in the treatment of cancer) by the name of George Blumenschein. It is probably unfair for me to single out one man when there were so many men and women who tried desperately to save my sister's life. But Dr. Blumenschein represented an attitude and spirit in medicine that we had not seen up until this point. Before coming to M. D. Anderson, her treatment had always been unilateral, meaning one doctor and one patient. Now, for the first time, Suzy was part of a team. *Dr. Blumenschein and his associates made Suzy a partner in every decision.* They were completely and totally honest with her and all of us about her condition. When Suzy arrived in Houston, she was a Stage IV cancer patient. This means that the disease had spread to other organs in her body and was still growing. It is a very critical situation. Dr. Blumenschein threw the book at her, in a sense. He not only told her everything, but he showed her the results of her tests. Rather than speak to Suzy in terms like "I will do this" or "I will do that," he said, "We can do this" or "Let's try that." He told Suzy exactly what her chances of survival were and what *they* had to do in order to fight this cancer. He said, "Susan, we will do everything we can to try to save you, but we can't do it without your help and cooperation." Suzy was not only *allowed* to ask questions, she was *encouraged* to do so.

Dr. Blumenschein's approach to the disease was an aggressive one. After recommending removing the lesion from her lung, he told Suzy that she had a 25-percent chance of survival, but that if she wouldn't give up, *he* wouldn't give up. He wanted to put her in a treatment protocol (that is, a combination of drugs—in this case the combination was being tested in a clinical trial) at M. D. Anderson and promised her that if one didn't work he would try another. Thus began a saga of intense chemotherapy. Chemotherapy is usually a combination of several drugs given together, delivered into the patient's bloodstream, that are highly toxic to fast-growing cells. The problem with chemotherapy is that it doesn't know the difference between the good guys and the bad guys, so a lot of important healthy cells are killed in the process, including the cells of the stomach lining and hair roots. Chemotherapy is often accompanied by nausea, mouth sores, hair thinning, and sometimes total hair loss, depending on the type used. (However, today there are very effective new drugs, which can relieve many of these side effects.) Suzy experienced all of that and more. Everyone given chemotherapy is warned that a side effect is hair loss, but nothing can prepare a woman for the shock and embarrassment of baldness. She bore up under the strain with all the dignity and grace she could manage, although I know she was devastated. Little did I know that even then, my sister was teaching me.

Her partnership with George Blumenschein gave Suzy focus. Because chemotherapy and radiation are given in cycles so that a patient can have alternate periods of treatment and rest, she was able to come home and spend time with her family between trips to Houston. While at home she tried to live as normal a life as possible, with the exception of a surgery to remove a small portion of her right lung where the cancer had invaded. She continued her charity work and spent long afternoons at the hospital in Peoria sitting with terminally ill patients. To this day I hear from the families of the people Suzy sat with. She even continued her modeling when she felt up to it, sporting a new look with a short-cut wig. She had sores in her mouth from all the medication, her arm was painful and swollen from lymphedema, and she had put on weight from the steroids used to slow her cancer, but Suzy still looked beautiful. I don't think I was ever more proud of my sister.

My mother, Stan, and I tried our best to be with her while she was in Houston. If we all couldn't be there together, one of us would be there at all times. She never went alone. There was a hotel apartment across the street from the medical center where patients stayed during their courses of chemotherapy and radiation. Besides being a lot less expensive than staying every night in the hospital, it gave the patient a little bit of freedom. On nights when Suzy wasn't feeling too sick, we were able to get out to eat or catch a movie. She was able to receive her second course of chemotherapy through what is called a Gershon or subclavian catheter. For her, it was a more comfortable way of receiving the drugs. The catheter is placed in a vein just above the clavicle and remains there throughout the course. A small battery-operated pump, which is carried by the patient either around the shoulder or on a belt, automatically delivers the chemo into the vein. You see, she couldn't receive the chemotherapy in the arm on the side of her surgery; there is too high a risk of infection. In the other arm, Suzy's veins had already collapsed from the continual abuse of so many needles.

When she wasn't in Houston I would visit Suzy in Peoria whenever I could. I was divorced by this time, living with my son, Eric. He was just a little boy of four then and was confused as to why I was gone so much. I tried to explain that his Aunt Suzy was very sick and needed me with her. I felt better for having always told Eric the truth, but I know it was a difficult period for him. It was a difficult time for everyone who knew and loved Suzy.

The stress and tension put on a family involved in a serious illness is unimaginable. You know you must stick together on the crucial matters, so often the tension released is by arguing about the little things. My father had a terrible time. He could not bear the sight of his precious daughter being so ill. Like many men of his generation, it was not easy for Dad to express his feelings openly. It was impossible for him to accept the fact that in this case he was not the one in control. As a result, it was our dear mother who bore the brunt of much of the burden. At one point she stayed in Houston for five and a half weeks without ever seeing the outside of the hospital. She wouldn't have it any other way. Fortunately, Mom had the strength to go it alone.

It was especially difficult for her because during this time the lumps in my breasts kept reappearing. I had my left breast biopsied three different times during Suzy's ordeal. Once she had to leave Suzy's side in Houston in order to be with me in Dallas. All three of my tumors were benign (noncancerous). I hated to worry my mother, but the truth is, I was scared. Every time I felt the slightest little abnormality, my heart began to race. I had learned that women whose mothers or sisters have had breast cancer have as much as two to three times the usual risk of developing the disease.

Whenever we felt as if we couldn't go on, that the load was just too heavy, it was Suzy's grace and humor that got us through the day. She was able to find something to smile about with every turn of the road and her infectious, warm concern was felt throughout the hospital.

The one thing Suzy never found humor in, however, was the aesthetic conditions of the waiting rooms. The walls were empty, the chairs uncomfortable, and sometimes a patient would have to sit there waiting six or more hours for a scheduled appointment. Suzy was horrified and so was I. She was more concerned with the treatment of the patients while my concern was the treatment of the disease. I was outraged that more hadn't been learned to help my sister. "Nan," she said, "as soon as I get better, let's do something about this. You can find a way to speed up the research. I know you can. And I want to fix up this waiting room and make it pretty for the women who have to be here. This isn't right."

For about fifteen months the Houston team of Blumenschein, his associates, and Komen were successful in slowing down her breast cancer. But then, for reasons known only to God, the disease started to rage inside her once again. Fully aware of her condition, but never willing to give up or talk about it, Suzy began a perilous and painful downhill battle. There was more surgery and more chemotherapy, but by now her body had built up a resistance to the drugs. Her cancer had gotten so out of control that it broke through the skin, resulting in grotesque sores all over her chest. Her breast implant had to be replaced with some muscle from her back to restore the chest area. Plastic surgery after plastic surgery to cover up these lesions was performed. She also had an operation called an oophorectomy, which is the removal of the ovaries. In some cases an oophorectomy has been proven quite successful in slowing down the growth of the disease because certain types of breast cancer feed off female hormones. In some cases—but not Suzy's. She began to spend more time feeling awful and we spent more time feeling helpless. None of us knew what to do anymore. Up until this point we had always spoken enthusiastically about our future together. It was becoming more obvious with each new day that this *was* our future with Suzy.

I remember one afternoon at M. D. Anderson, we were walking from the hospital over to the hotel. Suzy had just been through an awful experience. Her lungs had started to fill with fluid and I watched as nearly a gallon of fluid was drained from them to keep her from drowning. It was very painful for her and I could barely stand to hear her gasping for breath. The street we had to cross was quite a busy one, and as we waited for the light to change I saw a large bus barreling our way just about to pass where Suzy and I were standing. For a split second I contemplated the thought of how much easier it would be on her if she were to *accidentally fall* in front of that bus and end it all. I remembered her saying to me a long time ago that if she ever had to go through what Aunt Rose went through that she would want me to find a way to kill her. She'd rather be dead. I'm sure many of us have had similar thoughts, but when it actually happens the will to live becomes much stronger than anything else in the world. I wanted my sister with me for as long as possible *regardless* of the circumstances. *But the reality of the situation is that it really can get that bad.*

Another afternoon during the time when Suzy stayed in Houston, we were lying together by the pool at the hotel. She loved to sunbathe as often as possible, because she felt that having color on her face was the only thing that made her look healthy. As I watched her lying there reading, I took note of her thin, frail body and strained breathing. Fortunately, Suzy was *into* her book and paid no attention to me. Had she looked over, she would have seen my tears and known immediately what I was thinking. Our time together was drawing to a close. In a flood of beautiful memories I began to look back on the sacred relationship I shared with my sister. Frantically, I wrote my memories down, fearing somehow I might forget one later. I didn't realize then that memories so special are never forgotten. I also didn't realize that what I was writing that sunny afternoon was my sister's eulogy.

In quiet desperation, my parents, Stan, and I went to Suzy and Stan's rabbi for advice. He told us not to give up encouraging Suzy to keep trying but that under no circumstances were we to lie to her. It was time to begin saying our good-byes. Our family had always been totally honest with each other, and breaking that trust at this point would hurt Suzy much more than help her. Shortly after that discussion I was home in Peoria visiting one evening. My parents and Stan had taken Scott and Stephanie out to dinner and Suzy and I were home alone. She had just come back from Houston after an intense dose of chemo. I could hear her being violently ill in the bathroom. Throughout her three-year illness, Suzy was very brave and always maintained a great deal of pride in her appearance. I knew she preferred to be left alone at times like this. But on that particular night she just kept getting sicker and sicker and pretty soon I couldn't take it anymore. I ran into the bathroom and held her in my arms. "Oh, Nan," she sobbed, "isn't this awful? Don't I look horrible?"

"Yes, Suzy, it is horrible," I cried with her. "I can't imagine why this is happening to you."

After my sister was released from M. D. Anderson, I tried to come home every other week for a visit. Although she was too weak to get out of the car, Suzy insisted on riding with my parents to and from the airport when I came into town. Even though she could do little more than lie there in the back seat, this was her way of saying that she was still capable of taking care of me and that she was still there for me if I needed her. I did.

One particular Sunday afternoon on the way back to the airport, Suzy spoke to me again about doing something to help the sick women in the hospital. This practically tore my heart out because here she was, hardly able to manage a whisper, and she was worrying about other people. I couldn't bear it. When my father pulled up to the curb, I quickly kissed them both good-bye and jumped out of the car. I was just about inside the airport when I heard a funny sound that sounded like my name. I stopped in my tracks and turned around. There was Suzy, standing up outside the car on wobbly knees, wig lightly askew. With her arms outstretched, she said gently, "Good-bye, Nanny. I love you." I hugged her so hard I was afraid she might crumble. And then I ran to catch my plane.

I never saw my sister alive again. After nine operations, three courses of chemotherapy, and radiation, she had lost her three-year war. By the time I flew back to her side it was too late. She was gone.

Mother and I went to the funeral home to say a final farewell in private before her services began. When I approached Suzy, lying there so peacefully, I was shocked when I got close enough to see her face. My shock quickly changed to fury. Whoever had applied her makeup must have been the only person in Peoria who didn't know my sister. Her face looked overly made-up and phony, not at all like the soft, gentle woman we all loved so dearly. I insisted they remove all the makeup from her face at once. And then, alone, with my own cosmetics, I reapplied her makeup the way she had taught me to do so many years before. Mom sat off to the side and just watched, while silent tears rolled down her cheeks.

The months after Suzy's funeral were the saddest in my life. I wanted to stay near my parents because I knew they needed me (the truth is, we needed each other), but I had a son and a home that had been without any attention for a long time. It was time to get on with it, to pick myself up and start living again. I owed that to Eric. Some things are easier said than done.

I spent a lot of time thinking about Suzy. There is no way to accurately describe the void her absence left in my life. I also spent a great deal of time questioning my faith and wondering why such a good person was taken from a family that needed her so desperately. I often wondered, as many people do when they've lost a loved one, what really happens to a soul when a person dies. Was Suzy watching me? Did she hear me when I called her name out loud? After much thought I came to the conclusion that I would never know until I died myself, but I sure as hell didn't want to die in order to find out. Just in case, I wanted to do something to let her know how special she would always be in my heart. I was haunted by our last conversation and lay awake sometimes all night wondering what I could do to help other women with breast cancer. *Could one person really make a difference?*

CHAPTER TWO

My Story

A t a time when I needed a friend more than anything else in my life, in November of 1980, I met a man named Norman Brinker. Norman was and still is an extremely successful businessman in Dallas. I knew he was an eligible bachelor and had seen him at several charity functions in the city. What I had no way of knowing about was the depth of his

> *...love is the only thing that we can carry with us when we go, and it makes the end easy.*
>
> LOUISA MAY ALCOTT

character and the quality of his spirit. Norman isn't like any of the men I had previously met. He isn't at all interested in power. That's not to say he doesn't have any; he's enormously powerful. But he doesn't have to make other people look bad to make himself look good. Subjugation isn't Norman's style. He's a lover of people and a lover of life. I don't think he's ever met a person he didn't learn something from. He listens. There is a calmness about Norman that is a great balance for me.

From our first conversation, we knew we had a special bond. Norman had been married to tennis star Maureen (Little Mo) Connolly, and lost her to ovarian cancer in 1969. He, more than anyone else, understood my loss. We could talk about anything and everything, and we did. Norman taught me to laugh again, something for which I will never be able to thank him adequately. What seemed like a whirlwind courtship to most of our friends seemed perfectly right to us. We had a great deal in common, including our love of horses, skiing, and politics. Norman and I married on Valentine's Day in 1981.

But for all my happiness and contentment as Norman's wife, I still wanted to do something about Suzy's dream. I wanted to fulfill the pledge we had made about the way women with breast cancer were treated and try to make the country more aware of its devastating statistics. I didn't have the faintest idea where to begin. Norman pointed out that I had had a great deal of fundraising experience for a number of different charities. He suggested that I put that energy into the cause that was now so dear to my heart. Of course—I would start a charitable fund for breast cancer research. Norman was very supportive of this idea and said: "Sure, it's okay with me, but please don't call my friends." Of course, the next day I went right out and started calling them.

Breast cancer, I had learned the hard way, was the second-leading killer of women in the United States. Yet, even in 1981, it was not easy to discuss the disease publicly. I was very sure that most of my friends had no idea that over one hundred thirty-eight thousand new cases of the disease were detected every year, or that in 1940 one in twenty women were diagnosed with the disease but in 1981 the figure was one in thirteen. Throughout my sister's three-year illness, I had learned a lot about breast cancer, but I knew that if I expected people in Dallas to reach into their pockets, I'd better know a lot more about the disease scientifically. I studied with a vengeance. I called the National Cancer Institute and asked them to send me everything they could on the disease, and I read it. All of it. For a while, I'm sure I was an unwelcome guest at parties. I couldn't help myself. If a conversation started off about politics or child care, I'd somehow manage to turn it around to mammography and mastectomy. I not only found the statistics of breast cancer horrifying, I was shocked at how little people knew or seemed to *want* to know about this enemy. The subject made people extremely squeamish, especially men. If it weren't such a serious matter, I would have been amused. They can talk about war with no problem. Murder is interesting. Bankruptcy is fascinating. But breast cancer? Next subject. I've always had the feeling that women's breasts were an easy topic of contemplation for men among themselves or in the bedroom, but discussing them with women in a dignified manner was a different story altogether.

Yes, I had my work cut out for me. It was clear that I had to gain the interest and support of women in order to get my project off the ground. It was also clear that this was an undertaking that could not be managed by one person. Together with a few friends who had, through personal experiences, a similar passion for the cause, I began my unending race for the cure of breast cancer. At this point, exactly what the "project" was, was still undefined. All we had were our hearts in the right places, two hundred dollars in cash, a borrowed typewriter, and a shoe box.

By the end of 1983, with a lot of hard work and a great deal of luck, we had turned that two hundred dollars into one hundred fifty thousand dollars (today it is estimated the foundation has raised $39 million dollars). Former First Lady Betty Ford had graciously joined our efforts and was actively involved in helping to make the country more aware of the disease. Because of her influence over my sister and the bravery and strength she exuded throughout her own battle with breast cancer, we established the Betty Ford Award in her honor. This award is given annually, by Mrs. Ford herself, to the person whose contribution in the area of breast cancer research or education is most significant. Additionally, we established several other monetary awards to nurture promising treatment breakthroughs throughout the country. As our organization grew, we saw the need to establish an endowment to ensure our future, thus becoming the Susan G. Komen Breast Cancer Foundation. As our reputation grew, we began receiving requests for help from some of the most respected researchers in America. I cannot begin to explain the thrill of seeing our efforts make a difference.

One cold night in January 1984, Norman and I had just gotten into bed and I was pulling the comforter up over us in an attempt to get warm, when purely by accident and without any forewarning, as my hand skimmed lightly over my chest, I felt a small, hard lump in my left breast. I sprang out of bed, screaming, "Oh my God, I have a lump!" Norman told me to calm down, to call M. D. Anderson in the morning and fly to Houston to have it checked out. If it hadn't been close to midnight, I would have gone right then. At the crack of dawn the next morning, I had Fred Ames on the phone. Fred is a surgeon at M. D. Anderson whom I had asked to monitor my breasts. I had become somewhat of a case study in Houston because of the family history as well as my own history of benign breast tumors. I had immense respect for Dr. Ames's work and a high regard for him personally. I told him this lump felt different from the others and that I was very concerned. He said for me to get on the next plane and come right down.

After feeling my breast and reviewing my mammogram, Dr. Ames said, "Nancy, I don't think it's anything to worry about. I really feel like it is another benign tumor. I hate for you to keep having this breast biopsied because it has been done three times already and you've got so much scar tissue now, it is going to be difficult to see what we've got in there. Let's watch it for just a little while and see if it changes."

Well, I took his advice and went back to Dallas. I knew Dr. Ames had good logical and medical reasoning behind his decision. But I had become an expert in the normal changes of my own breasts, and I knew *this lump felt different.* The other three had felt rubbery and this one was very hard.

The next day the foundation was sponsoring a seminar on breast cancer detection. As you entered the room where the seminar was to take place, there were display tables set up with all kinds of written material for the guests to take with them. There were also several breast forms with hidden lumps in them so that the women could come by and feel exactly what we were talking about. As I stood there welcoming our guests, my hand fell behind me absently and I unconsciously began to feel the forms. Surprisingly enough, I had never done this before. I came across something that felt a little too familiar. One of the lumps in the form felt very much like the one in my own breast. As I stood in front of that group of women speaking about how important it is to be vigilant about your breast health, I wondered what they would say if they knew that at that very moment I thought I had a serious problem.

After the seminar I went to see my surgeon here in Dallas, Morris Fogelman. Dr. Fogelman had removed my previous three lumps and really knew my history. He was aware of the fact that I had since become a case study at M. D. Anderson, but I had always been very comfortable with him and just wanted another opinion. He said, "Nancy, that does not feel good to me, and if I were you, I'd get it out." I didn't want to overreact, and I had to take into consideration that Dr. Fogelman had said the same thing about my other three lumps, but I had a feeling he was right. He took me upstairs and did a test called transillumination (also known as diaphonography), which involves shining a bright light through the breast to illuminate its interior. Different types of tissues transmit and scatter the light in different ways. The test is read on an infrared-sensitive television camera. Studies indicate that transillumination, however, is unable to detect the tinier lumps routinely found in mammography. I felt the test was unnecessary for me. Although it was and still is effective in finding large lumps, I already knew I had a lump and wasn't looking for confirmation. What I wanted to know was whether or not I had cancer. Unfortunately, that can only be determined at this point by a biopsy or needle biopsy. Still, the radiologist who read the test said he, too, felt that my tumor was benign because it was a very round lump with clear definition all the way around it. The name cancer is derived from a Latin word meaning crab. When you picture a crab in your mind, its claws and legs reach out away from its body. The disease cancer is thought to do the same thing. It often spreads out in all directions, invading the healthy tissues and organs of the body. That is why having a perfectly round, clearly defined lump can be a good sign.

Once again, I went home and on about my business. There probably wasn't one waking fifteen-minute time span that I went without poking and feeling that lump. I swore to myself I could feel it growing. Ten days later I went back to Dr. Fogelman. He said, "Nancy, it *is* getting bigger; get it out of there." Immediately, I called Fred Ames and told him I wanted this thing out—no matter what it was. He said, "No problem. Come on down—we'll do it here in the office. I feel very confident about it's being benign, but I know you're troubled so let's get rid of it. I'll give you a local anesthetic and do a biopsy right here in my office."

Norman was in Florida on business and my parents were also in Florida where they spend most of the winter. I called and told them I was going to Houston but that Dr. Ames felt sure there was nothing to worry about and that my friend Sandy would accompany me to the hospital. I made everyone feel I was not nervous, but the truth is I had a very uneasy feeling in the pit of my stomach.

Sandy and I were greeted at M. D. Anderson by Doris Bechtold, one of the patient-care coordinators at the hospital, a woman who had treated me and my family as her own from the first day we brought Suzy in the door. Dr. Ames brought me right into the day surgery room. I was given a local anesthetic so that I was completely awake and alert. A short curtain was placed directly under my chin so that I couldn't see the actual surgery, but I stared into Fred Ames's eyes for the entire operation searching for a clue. He didn't give me one. When a biopsy is done the suspicious tissue is mounted and sent to the pathology department for analysis. Some of the tissue is frozen and mounted on a slide for an immediate microscopic examination. Through the examination of the "frozen section," results can be determined in a matter of minutes. Analyzing the "permanent section" of the tissue can take several days. I wanted my results as quickly as possible, so I asked for both. I was wheeled into the recovery room where I waited for what seemed like an hour or more. All of a sudden, Dr. Ames burst through the door. I looked up at him and said, "Another false alarm, right?"

He said, "No, Nancy, it's not. It's cancer."

I remember leaping off the bed and screaming, "Tell me you're not telling me this! Tell me you're kidding! Please tell me what you're saying is not the truth!" And then I sobbed.

He walked over, hugged me, and said quietly, "Nancy, I sent it back twice because I didn't want to believe the diagnosis, but it is confirmed. You've got cancer. Now, I want you to calm down. It was very small and I think we've gotten it very early. You have a lot of options."

I just remember screaming, "I want them both off today. Get them off me! I want them off now!" I was so scared and so angry and so upset.

Fred told me to get dressed, call Norman and my mother, and then we would talk about the situation rationally. Well, I couldn't reach Norman, but I did reach my mother. She said that she would get Norman and they would both be there on the next flight. All I could think of was Suzy. I remembered how she didn't

want a mastectomy and how desperately afraid I was of following in her footsteps. My mom asked me what I wanted to do, and
I told her to get rid of both breasts. Then I talked with Fred and
he said he really didn't feel that was necessary. So, without another thought I said I wanted to get rid of the left breast for sure. As
soon as possible. I was aware, even then, of a procedure called
"lumpectomy," which was finally receiving the appropriate
amount of attention and approval it deserved through many
years of exhaustive study by a physician named Bernard Fisher.
A lumpectomy is a surgical procedure in which only the cancerous tumor is removed. It is usually followed by radiation and
sometimes other forms of *adjuvant therapy* (treatment other
than surgery). When a lumpectomy is a clinically viable option, it
saves a woman from losing her breast. Unfortunately, my tumor
was located very close to the nipple, making it difficult to get to
without totally disfiguring my breast. The cosmetic advantages
of a lumpectomy, in my case, did not apply. I knew that if I could
get through this alive, down the road I would have reconstructive
surgery. To be honest, how I would end up looking was not a priority at the time. I simply didn't want to die.

I checked myself into the hospital right away and went
through a whole battery of other tests. They did a full body X ray,
a bone survey, and another chest X ray to see if the cancer had
metastasized to other areas of my body. Doris Bechtold and Fred
Ames never left my side. All the tests came out negative, but I
couldn't allow myself to relax because I knew my lymph nodes
hadn't been tested yet and wouldn't be until surgery the next day.
George Blumenschein was away on a ski vacation. It would have
been a comfort to have had him there.

By the time my mother and Norman arrived that evening, I
was sedated, wailing, frightened, and confused. Both of them
looked me in the eye and said they *knew* I'd be all right. I wanted to believe it and in a way I could see myself well again. Still, I

couldn't afford to be too optimistic. Breast cancer is serious. The mental picture of Suzy at the end of her life, so small, shriveled, and weak, was haunting me. I was ready to fight and I wanted to get on with it. But that night I just wanted to be cuddled because the next day I was declaring war. Mother spent the night with me in the hospital. My breast burned from the biopsy, but I kept touching it anyway, thinking it would be the last time I'd be able to feel any sensation at all on that side of my chest. I thought about Eric and how frightened he must be. I thought about Norman and knew, although he'd never say, how frightened *he* must be after already having lived through the loss of one wife with cancer. And then I looked over at my mother, so brave and cheerful in the next bed. What must she be thinking? Was she preparing herself psychologically to lose another daughter after a long and gruesome illness? She seemed not to be. When she looked at me and said I would be fine, I searched her eyes for signs of untruth or pity. There were none.

The next thing I remember is being wheeled into the operating room the following morning. I touched my breast one more time before going under, and then it was over. When I was wheeled back to my room, it was filled with people and flowers. I went to sleep feeling loved, calm, and content to be alive.

It must have been the anesthesia, because that contented feeling certainly didn't last. The next morning I woke up wanting to get going, to do whatever it was that had to be done in order to get well. Dr. Ames came to see me and said that although my nodes looked clear to him, the official results wouldn't be back for a couple of days. He also told me that he had made the incision in a place where reconstruction would be easy should I decide to have it down the road. I couldn't see anything at that point because my entire chest was bandaged down to my waist. With all those bandages I couldn't even tell that one of my breasts was missing. What I felt was a hot, burning sensation all over my chest. There were tubes protruding from the wrapping on my left side to allow the excess fluid to be drained from my body. It is the body's natural response to automatically send fluid to a vacant pocket of flesh. At first there is too much fluid to be reabsorbed naturally, so the tubes are usually left in place for approximately three or four days.

I wasn't in pain; I guess this is where the term *uncomfortable* comes in to play. Mostly I was restless. I wanted to *do* something. My family and friends were babying me, treating me like a sick person—and I didn't feel sick. The first moment I was alone, I got out of bed and took a walk through the hospital and upstairs to the physical therapy room. I knew exactly where it was because I had been there with Suzy. I got on a stationary bike and was able to pedal a couple of miles before one of my nurses found me and demanded I get back in bed. I looked around at the other patients exercising and thought how bored they all looked. There was a precious little boy in the room who couldn't have been more than three years old. My heart ached for this little boy. I looked at his lost little face and thought about how unfair it was that he couldn't be outdoors playing with other little boys. I thought about how Suzy would have reacted if she had seen him. It would have broken her heart.

Anyone who has had cancer or knows anyone who has had cancer or has even read anything about people with cancer will hear one thing over and over again: This is a disease that makes a person feel completely out of control. When you get a cold or the flu you can usually feel it coming on. You know the probable outcome and you can prepare for it if not avoid it. But cancer is something you can't prepare for. By the time you know you've got it, the disease has quietly invaded your body without warning. There are things I did in an effort to take control of my body which I am sure other people would not choose to do. Remember, I was a very well-educated cancer patient at the time and I had seen the disease at its worst. But nothing could have prepared me for the shock and fear of discovering breast cancer in my own body. I thought I understood it because I was so close to Suzy, but in truth, I didn't. Each case is special. It comes with its own set of specifics, both medical and emotional. All I was certain of was that I would do *anything* I could to rid myself of this breast cancer and get on with my life.

George Blumenschein was at my side within a couple of days following my surgery. He had spoken to Fred Ames, and seen my lab reports, and, as is typically Blumenschein, gave it to me straight—chapter and verse. He said:

"Nancy, I think you are in a good situation. There was no node involvement and your tumor was still small. I feel very optimistic about your case, but I am going to recommend we treat this very aggressively for a number of reasons. First of all, your age. As a rule, the younger the patient, the more aggressive the cancer. Thirty-six is young to have breast cancer. And while your tumor was not wildly aggressive, it showed signs of being on the aggressive side, which can mean rapid growth. We also have to take into consideration the fact that your hormone receptor assay was negative [a hormone receptor assay is a test done at the time of biopsy to determine whether or not a breast cancer's growth is influenced by female hormones]. Today tamoxifen may also be prescribed as adjuvant therapy. And your previous family history with the disease is very important. I want to bring you from an 85-percent survival rate to a 95-percent survival rate. And for that I recommend four courses of chemotherapy to begin as soon as possible, right after your surgery heals."

He went on to explain that if I agreed to this form of treatment, I would lose all my hair and possibly experience other unpleasant side effects. Some people develop leukemia from chemotherapy; sometimes the hair doesn't grow back all the way. Some people get violently sick from the drugs, while others make it through the treatments with a minimal amount of discomfort.

Dr. Blumenschein assigned me to a protocol—a combination of drugs—being used in a clinical trial he was conducting at M. D. Anderson. I would be given several forms of chemotherapy including Adriamycin, 5-Fluorouacil (also known as 5-FU), and Cytoxan. In Part Two, chapter 6, I will explain more about these and other forms of chemotherapy, but for now what is important to know is that this is a high dosage of drugs intended to kill off fast-growing cells aggressively. Dr. Blumenschein also explained to me that since Suzy's illness, improvements had been made in the subclavian catheter and pump. He said I could be very mobile if I chose this method of drug delivery and that there was a class available at M. D. Anderson where I could learn everything I needed to know about administering the drugs myself in the safest way possible. I did take the class and I did have the catheter surgically implanted. All I could think about was survival. According to Dr. Blumenschein, I could increase my chances of survival by 10 percent. That's all I needed to hear. I wanted to go home to Eric and Norman and give them the mother and wife they had counted on. At the time, nothing else mattered.

I am a lucky woman. I had the means to get the best medical treatment available. And I was educated enough to know how to find it. Still, there were those who didn't agree with the treatment I chose. Some highly respected members of the medical community thought perhaps the treatment I agreed to was *too* aggressive. Maybe I didn't need a modified radical mastectomy; a lumpectomy would have been equally as effective. Maybe I didn't need such a strong dosage of chemotherapy. What the outcome would have been with a less aggressive treatment, I will never know, but to those who think I should have handled it differently, all I can offer in a way of explanation is this: The informed decision was mine to make. I was fully aware of all my options. Between Fred Ames and George Blumenschein I had a medical team I believed in. I trusted their advice, but that's what it was, advice. I had to do what I felt was right for me. It was funny because when Suzy was so sick, I looked at her and thought to myself, *I could never go through this. I could never voluntarily choose to submit my body to such torture.* But when push came to shove and I was faced with the same life-threatening disease, the choices were not difficult.

Besides having medical options and much more education, I was lucky in other ways which proved to be equally as important. I had good friends and a lot of people depending on me to get better. I had built the Susan G. Komen Breast Cancer Foundation not only in the hope of one day finding a cure, but with the intention of helping women make informed decisions about their own breast health. I not only wanted to fight this disease, I *had* to fight this disease the best way I knew how. My reputation depended on it. This is not to say that I recommend my form of treatment to anyone else. Each woman has to decide for herself which options best serve her needs. She has to assemble her own team of medical experts and make her informed decisions based on their advice.

My team consisted of more than medical experts. I had a strong support team of emotional and spiritual members as well. I don't know what I would have done without my mother's help. She was with me every step of the way, and still is to this day. Norman convinced me that he would love me exactly the same with or without both breasts. I had friends who kept me laughing throughout the whole ordeal, which could have been, perhaps, the best medicine of all. One friend, Barbara Hyde, who was being treated for breast cancer at the same time as Suzy, made an especially touching gesture. She came in one day and discreetly placed something in the drawer by my bed. There were other friends in the room when she was leaving so she whispered softly in my ear that I would need what she left when it came time to leave the hospital. As soon as I was alone, I looked in the drawer and saw that she had given me a prosthesis. A prosthesis is a breast form, in this case a bra with one side filled with artificial substances that I wore after my mastectomy to look "normal" in my clothes. I was very touched by Barbara's thoughtfulness and appreciative of her sensitivity in not mentioning it in front of anyone else.

One afternoon shortly after my surgery, I found myself alone in the room quietly contemplating my future. The phone next to my bed rang and it was Betty Ford. She wanted to know how I was doing. Immediately I began to fight back the tears. The more she spoke, the more emotional I became. I was embarrassed and told her so. I will never forget her words. She said:

"Nancy, allow yourself the luxury of tears. Cry your heart out and say all those things you're feeling. Really pity yourself and ask, 'Why me?' You need to do all of that...but only for one day. Get it all out of your system and then release it. Let it go. You have studied this disease like no one else. You know what you have to do. Trust yourself and believe in your good judgment. Try to get through one day at a time. If one day seems too overwhelming, try to get through it one hour at a time. The rest is up to God, whatever 'God' means to you. There is a line from the twenty-third psalm that goes, 'Though I walk through the valley of the shadow of death...' Nancy, it says you walk *through it, it doesn't*

say you have to stop there. You have a whole lot of people who love you very much and are pulling for you to recover."

When I hung up the phone, I took Mrs. Ford's advice and cried my heart out. I cried for Suzy and for Eric and for my parents and for Norman. I cried for myself. The next day I checked out of the hospital. It was time to start taking control. I didn't go straight home. My mother and I went wig shopping. Within my community, the word had spread like wildfire that I had cancer. I was already being called for radio and television interviews to discuss my disease and how I was planning to handle it. I thought the better I looked, the more positive the message I would be sending out. Immediately upon my return from the hospital, I went to my own hairdresser and had him cut my hair very short. The wigs I had purchased were of short styles, and I wanted the transition to look as smooth as possible.

This is something I had to do for me. It wasn't as if no one knew my hair was going to fall out. Of course, everyone I was close to knew what was happening. It was more a matter of preserving my dignity. I didn't want to give people any more reason to pity me. Letting myself go would have been, in my eyes, a form of surrendering to the disease. I was determined to stay on top of the situation as much as possible.

It was also very important to me to look good for Norman and Eric. Poor little Eric was so frightened. All he knew was that his Aunt Suzy had had breast cancer and she died. Now his mother had the same disease. He didn't understand the fact that mine was detected and treated much earlier than Suzy's or that my tumor was much smaller and not nearly as aggressive. At eight years old, none of that mattered to him. Norman was so sweet and kind and loving to me, but I didn't want him to think for one minute that just because Maureen had died, I would, too. Her death was the most painful thing he had ever experienced and I wanted him to know that I was very much alive and intended to stay that way. She was taken from Norman just as his first chain of restaurants, Steak and Ale, was becoming successful. Now that his second chain of restaurants, Chili's, was enjoying the beginning of what would become enormous success, I sure didn't want to give my husband anything more to worry about. I also knew that my appearance was going to get worse before it got better. Remember, at this point, I was still all bandaged up, so he had yet to see his single-breasted wife. And although my hair had been cut very short, it was still *my* hair. No, the best thing I could do for the men in my life was convince them I felt well. That meant makeup, wigs when the time came, and the best general appearance I could possibly muster.

My mother volunteered to come back to M. D. Anderson for the four courses of chemotherapy. I felt awful to be putting her through the same hell she knew all too well, but she insisted. To be honest, I couldn't think of anyone else I'd rather have with me. I also knew what was ahead and it would be difficult to convince Norman I was well if he saw how sick the treatment was bound to make me. He had taught me to smile again, a few years back, and I wanted to make sure, now, that he kept smiling.

Like Suzy, I was not confined to the hospital. For the first part of the treatment I received a combination of 5-FU and Cytoxan delivered through an IV drip directly into the subclavian catheter. That was followed by four days of continuous infusion of Adriamycin through a small pump. I was given four vials of the drug to take with me over to the hospital hotel. As each of the vials emptied into the catheter a little signal went off to let me know it was time to make the change. It was kind of a tricky procedure because the catheter has to be meticulously cleaned in order to prevent infection. I am not mechanically inclined at all and didn't enjoy fiddling with it. Mother was very helpful and made sure the job was done right. That night I felt pretty good, so Mom and I went out for dinner. I was in the mood for a juicy hamburger and fries, a treat I don't often allow myself. But I felt I deserved it, so we threw our diets to the wind and indulged. By the time we got to bed, I was content and tired, looking forward to a good night's sleep. It wasn't to be. At three o'clock in the morning I woke up violently ill, with the most wretched, flu-like symptoms you could imagine. I was ill over and over again until I began to dehydrate, and Mother took me right back to the clinic. They gave me an IV and Seven-Up or Gatorade with chipped ice. And they put me on an antinausea drug. (Today's drugs do not have as many side-effects.)

Suzy used to complain of having a metallic taste in her mouth after chemotherapy and now I knew what she meant. I became acutely sensitive to all kinds of smells—things that had never bothered me before could make me turn absolutely green. It was a ghastly experience, but before long I had finished my first round and was home again in Dallas. They sent me home with all kinds of antidepressants, Valium and who knows what else, to try to relieve some of the side effects of the chemo. I tried to take as little medicine as possible. I've never been one to take a lot of pills, and I wanted to save the drugs for times when I really needed them because I know your body can build up an immunity toward certain medications. For the first few days I felt mildly flu-like and then I started to feel good again. I got dressed every day and although I wasn't up for aerobics, I made it a personal goal to at least get out and walk, even if it was just for a short time.

I was very self-conscious the first time I got into bed with Norman. I didn't quite know what to do or what he would think. I shouldn't have worried. He made me believe that it really didn't matter that my left breast was missing. *I* was much more sensitive on the subject than he was.

Nine days after my first round of chemotherapy I was sitting in front of the mirror brushing my hair and felt it happening. I looked at the brush and it was filled with my little short hairs. I cannot explain the feeling that came over me. Suzy had tried to describe it, but I didn't fully understand until I experienced it myself. A huge wave of panic took over my whole body. It didn't matter that I knew it was coming or that I was prepared for it. The truth is, I don't think you can ever be *really* prepared for going bald. That first day I was probably the only one who noticed any difference at all. I was terrified of what Eric would think. I didn't want him to be afraid of me. The next day, it was even worse—lots more hair in the brush. I felt completely out of control, the disease was gaining on me. I was there alone in my room crying, feeling terribly sorry for myself. Then I remembered Mrs. Ford's encouraging words and realized I had already done my crying. It was time to get on with it. I had to get back in control. I stood up, got into a steaming hot shower, and finished the job myself. I yanked every hair out of my head before it could fall out on its own. Then I sat in front of the mirror again and stared and stared at my head from all angles until I was comfortable with the new me, or at least as comfortable as I would ever get. I wanted to deal with the situation and face the facts. *As a side effect to getting rid of my breast cancer, I was going to be temporarily bald.*

I did my best to keep my round, bald head covered up at all times. I wore scarves and turbans, and my wigs. As time went on, I became more relaxed about the hair thing, though I never went to bed bareheaded. Besides the obvious reason of wanting to look as appealing as possible to Norman, it should be duly noted that a bald head is a cold head. You have no idea unless you've been through it how cold your body can get without hair. And, just for the record, your head isn't the only place you lose it. I felt I looked more like a plucked chicken than a woman. Eric did walk in my bedroom once and see my head before I could get covered up, and I know he was really jolted. But that soon passed and before too long, he was back to acting like an eight-year-old boy. Sometimes when I was getting ready to leave the house, Eric would come over innocently to kiss me good-bye, and yank off my wig and run off with it. Naturally, I'd run after him screaming and soon we'd end up on the floor laughing until the tears streamed from our eyes. I was enormously grateful for those silly times because it proved that our relationship transcended the disease. I know I often took the anger I was feeling about being burdened with breast cancer out on Eric and Norman. It might have been a "normal" reaction, but it wasn't fair to them. They were, and are, so wonderful to me, I regret being robbed of even one moment of quality time together.

I went back to the Komen Foundation and resumed as many of my responsibilities as possible. As hard as I tried to look and feel good at home, I think I tried even harder at work. In my mind, I had to prove that I was the ideal cancer patient.

When April came, it was time for me to go back to Houston for Round Two. I had come up with another idea I was anxious to discuss with George Blumenschein. As much as I know the automatic pump is a remarkable device for many patients and that most people love it, I really didn't feel it was the best option for me. I realize that the pump allows patients their freedom to more or less continue with as normal a life as possible, but I am an impatient woman and wanted the whole thing over with yesterday. More important, I didn't like the idea of giving myself the medication. Quite frankly, I didn't really trust myself to do it right and I was tired of burdening my mother with the responsibility. What I wanted to do was check myself into M. D. Anderson and have Dr. Blumenschein put me to sleep, speed up the process of the delivery of the chemotherapy to two days, and be done with it. One night in the hospital, two days of treatment, and that's it.

We discussed this idea at great length. That's one of the things I loved and still love about George Blumenschein—he always treated me with great respect and considered my opinions. We were truly partners in my treatment. He understood my reasons for wanting my medication in this manner and had come to know my impatience as well as anyone. He explained that I couldn't be knocked out completely during chemotherapy because if I got sick from the medication I could easily choke, and also that the process could only be sped up so much. So we compromised. First, I turned in the pump I used for the initial course. I was allowed to be sedated but not asleep during the treatment. I did have four days' worth of chemo administered in two days' time through an IV drip. The catheter remained in my body for the IV, but I no longer had to fiddle with it except to keep the area clean and infection-free. The first time we tried this, it didn't go quite as smoothly as I had hoped. I still got pretty sick, but at least it was over a lot sooner. Today, thanks to a drug called Ondansetron, nausea is all but eliminated.

There was something about recuperating at home I found particularly comforting. Looking out of my own window at my own lawn gave me a feeling of inner peace. As I enjoyed the luxuries of home and family, my mind kept bringing me back to all the other women I had seen at M. D. Anderson who were not financially as fortunate. Breast cancer, like all deadly diseases, is expensive. What could the foundation do for these women? It was then, in the spring of 1984, that the idea of a low-cost screening center was born. This idea turned into reality in 1986 at Parkland Hospital in Dallas.

I did notice something unusual happening after my second course of chemotherapy: I was having awful "black dreams." I have since learned they are a common side effect, but I found them horrifying. I could never remember exactly what went on in the dreams but they were dark, mysterious, and ugly. I would wake in the night absolutely terrified. In order to go back to sleep I would wander into the kitchen and pour myself a glass of wine, or two. It was the first and only time I ever thought I was drinking too much. It wasn't that I was drinking huge quantities of alcohol, but two glasses of wine every day on top of the pills and chemotherapy was taking its toll on my body. We now know that a person undergoing chemotherapy should stay away from alcohol altogether. It is not good for the system to mix cytotoxic drugs and alcohol. I felt lethargic and overweight and irritable. The realization scared me to death. I cut out the wine for a long time and focused on a healthy diet and a regular exercise routine. I began to feel better and noticed I was regaining my strength faster. Much to my parents' displeasure, I even considered starting to ride horses again. I began to set small, achievable physical goals for myself, gearing up to one big goal which was to play in a polo match by the end of July. Norman was worried, too, but knew by now that once I had made up my mind he couldn't stop me. So he watched, and being a superb polo player himself, coached my riding and made sure I wasn't taking on too much too fast.

My third and fourth courses of chemotherapy went like clockwork. After a few minor adjustments in the combinations of the medicine, Dr. Blumenschein and I had found a way to make it work. It was, for me, a great accomplishment. The euphoria of completing chemotherapy was tempered, however, by a feeling of panic that I was no longer doing anything to fight the cancer. I was, of course, thrilled to be done with the treatment, but now what was I supposed to do? Sit back and do nothing? I couldn't help remembering when Suzy thought *she* was cured. Would that happen to me? It is a bevy of mixed emotions experienced by every cancer patient. The feeling is frightening, almost like the first day of school. You feel alone, timid, afraid to get back into the mainstream. I had been well taken care of by

George Blumenschein, my family, and my friends, and now it was time to fly solo again.

The only thing that kept me sane was following the advice of another friend and cancer expert, the late Rose Kushner. She had said, "Nancy, always keep a full calendar. Don't give yourself a chance to worry and don't ever plan for a time when you might not be around to fulfill all the obligations you have made."

These were wise words, ones that I have repeated often to other cancer patients. This advice, in addition to striving for a physical goal, kept me going through that most difficult time period. I had set the physical goal, which was to play in a polo match by July. It was now time to prove to my friends that I was back.

I threw myself into fund-raising for the Komen Foundation. My friend Carolyn Williams had been working furiously to organize a function we called "Race for the Cure." It was an auction with prizes of a masculine nature, the purpose of which was to heighten awareness and support for breast cancer from the men in Dallas. It worked. *That night alone the Komen Foundation raised almost one million dollars for breast cancer research.*

I started to ride every day and had begun swinging the polo mallet once again. The truth is, it felt great. Yes, I wore out easily, but I also felt invigorated and alive. When it came time to play in that match, I was ready. I am sure I was a sight for sore eyes. It probably wasn't fair of me to put the other players through what they had to observe, but there I was, bald as a billiard ball, charging down the field with nothing under my helmet but a scarf. My mother and father were standing on the side of the field with a small oxygen tank, of all things, in case of an emergency. It was a blazing hot July day in Dallas and I guess they were afraid I would pass out from the heat. Norman and Eric were also there, watching on the sidelines. Our team won the match, and afterward, when the photographs were taken, I was the only player who didn't remove her helmet—a gesture I am sure was greatly appreciated by all. The victory, for me, had little to do with polo. For the next year and a half I went through what my mother terms "the checkup crazies." My friend Carolyn Walker, also a former cancer patient, calls it "toe cancer." What it means is that every tiny ache or pain is immediately assumed to be the worst. You are torn between wanting to rush to the doctor every other minute and at the same time being scared to death to step into his office. Dr. Blumenschein had gone into private practice in Arlington, a city right outside of Dallas. I am sure I drove him nearly out of his mind, but he was always concerned, always ready and eager to see me.

It wasn't until almost two years after my initial surgery that I really started to look at myself and think about reconstruction. I was getting undressed for bed one night and happened to get a good look at my lopsided body in the mirror. I thought, *I really don't like this.* My parents and Norman were going to be spending a great deal of time in Florida on business, and I just didn't want to be operated on or recuperating in Texas when the people I depended on most were going to be on the East Coast. Although I am a knowledgeable cancer patient and like to think of myself as a strong woman, like anyone else, I want to be near people who make me feel safe when I'm not 100 percent well. My family does that for me.

After a lot of investigation, I went to a doctor by the name of John Bostwick in Atlanta, Georgia. Dr. Bostwick has published several textbooks on the subject, and he showed me dozens of pictures of his work. His latest book, *A Woman's Decision*, explains in complete detail the latest reconstruction procedures. He told me how he thought the surgery should be done and how it would probably turn out. He also told me about the risks and everything that could possibly go wrong. I liked him and respected him right away.

With Norman and Eric at high school graduation [1994]

With Norman

Eric, Mother, and Suzy's daughter,
Stephanie, at the tenth-year celebration
of the Komen Foundation (1992).
(Photo by J. Alan Hansley)

The operation was fairly easy. Dr. Bostwick simply reopened the scar left in exactly the right place by Dr. Ames and slid in a silicone implant underneath the skin and chest muscles. He did a little bit of mastopexy (reduction) on the other breast so that they would match. Six months later I had the nipple put on. He took a little piece of skin from my thigh and fashioned the whole nipple areola complex so that it pretty much looked the same as the other one.

For the first procedure I was in the hospital for a few days. The surgery was on Monday, and the following Sunday I was watching Norm's polo match in Dallas. I was aware of the implant being there, but my whole chest area was still largely numb.

I was extremely pleased with the results and on the day I went to the department store to purchase my first *real* bra again in two years, I felt as giddy as a thirteen-year-old. It was fun to wear clothes that showed cleavage; I had almost forgotten what it was like. There are other types of reconstruction available now (see chapter 7), and they should be reviewed with your physician to determine what is right for you. This was right for me at the time. Unfortunately, silicone implants have proven troublesome for many women. The Food and Drug Administration has removed them from the market except for limited usage. Saline implants are still approved for use, though there are challenges with these as well.

The one problem I had not anticipated was lymphedema, which is swelling and collection of fluid in the arm on the side of the mastectomy. I knew all about it, of course, but had gone to great lengths to prevent it from happening to me. I maintained a low-salt diet, exercised the arm regularly, and kept it free of jewelry. I was very careful and therefore, not the lymphedema prototype. But about a year after my reconstruction, I accidentally burned my arm on the stove. It became infected and the infection caused my arm to blow up like a balloon. It was grotesque. I don't remember ever being so mad. Here I had suffered through the cancer, endured chemotherapy, worn a prosthesis for two years, and had a great success with my reconstruction. I had done everything possible to look normal again, and now this.

Dr. George Peters, a Dallas breast surgeon, recommended a physical therapist, whom I saw every day. Some people told me that once an infection set in, the condition could be irreversible. George Blumenschein, too, had doubts about my recovery from lymphedema. But I wasn't going to accept it, not even from Blumenschein. As far as I was concerned, not making a complete recovery wasn't an option for me. I became even more emphatic about my diet, I exercised like a crazy person, wore an elastic sleeve on my arm all the time to try to bring the swelling down, and took antibiotics every day. Eventually, it worked, but the whole process took over a year. I am not sure that women are warned about lymphedema with enough urgency. It is a serious problem that, I feel, can disfigure a woman far more visibly than a mastectomy. To me, the mastectomy was easy to hide but when your entire arm, from the shoulder to the wrist, is three times the size of your other arm, now *that's* difficult to cover up. And the *last* thing a woman needs to hear is that it is an irreversible condition. I didn't accept that, and I don't think any woman should. You know, sometimes patients can teach their doctors a thing or two about medicine. George Blumenschein often talks about what I taught him on the subject of lymphedema. There have been improvements in the treatment of lymphedema since that time. Ask your physician for the latest treatments or combinations of treatments.

Although many have said it, it doesn't make the statement any less true: When you are told you have cancer, your life changes forever. *Forever.* I have always been a doer, always wanted to get things done yesterday. The long-term effect of having breast cancer for me has been to make me do everything in my life even faster.

I have no idea what tomorrow will bring so I don't wait for my future to run its course; I make it happen. I think it drives my family and friends crazy. Norman says I don't relax enough, that I push too hard. But I can't help it. There are a lot of things I want to get done while I'm healthy enough to do them. Subconsciously, perhaps I feel that if I slow down even for a short while, I am saying to those cancer cells, "Come and get me." Still, it doesn't do you any good to worry constantly about what *might* happen. That takes all the fun out of life. I have done everything I know that is possible to be healthy. I was beginning to have some very unpleasant female problems. The chemotherapy I received during treatment for breast cancer had altered my hormones and periods. My doctors felt that I needed estrogen regulation and that to give me estrogen would be inappropriate with my history of breast cancer—unless I had my ovaries removed. I decided to have a complete hysterectomy with oophorectomy (removal of ovaries). I am glad I did it. For me it was right. It might not be right for everyone. Some women do go on to have children after breast cancer, depending on the specifics of their disease. Given *my* family's history, I opted to forgo that possibility. The operation prevented me from having the one thing in life I might truly miss, a child with Norman. But we each have children, who together make our own family, which is more than some people *ever* have. For that I am thankful.

Now you know the whole story. I said I would tell you everything, and I have. Who knows what tomorrow will bring. At times throughout the years, it has seemed to me and the members of my family as if we were acting out parts in some unfathomable novel rather than participating in real life. Other times we have felt so much a part of *real life* that the energy surges through our bones like a bolt of lightning. There is more to this, however, than the trauma experienced by my family. The good news is all that has happened *because* of it. The thousands of women and the men who make up the Susan G. Komen Breast Cancer Foundation have made enormous strides in bringing public awareness of breast cancer to the forefront. The money we have raised has helped to fund a number of significant research projects. For example, it has gone to Johns Hopkins Oncology Center in Baltimore, Maryland, and the Vincent T. Lombardi Cancer Research Center in Washington, D.C., for the study of tumor growth factors; the National Cancer Institute in Bethesda, Maryland, for the study of how the disease progresses in the body; the MD Anderson Cancer Center in Houston, Texas, and The University of California at Berkeley to study genetics and breast cancer; Baylor University Medical Center in Dallas, Texas, for work in Magnetic Resonance Imaging (MRI) for early detection; University of Texas Health Science Center in San Antonio, Texas, for the study of the anti-cancer drug tamoxifen. Countless local education projects and low-cost, no-cost screening mammography programs have been funded as well.

We have also been successful in our attempt to change legislation in Texas so that insurance coverage for mammograms for women over the age of thirty-five is mandatory. We will not rest until similar laws are passed in all states. Foundation leaders testified on behalf of the 1992 Mammography Quality Standards Act passed by Congress requiring all mammography facilities and technicians to be certified by an accrediting body. My great friend Max Fisher, Republican statesman and Jewish leader, says, "Politics is the art of the possible." I believe him. To help make screening and mammography more accessible, we actively work with groups in the development of screening programs around the country. Thousands of women are screened each year in Susan G. Komen-funded programs nationwide. Our mobile screening vans service communities where there are no

National Cancer Institute and Komen Foundation Summit on Mammography, Washington, D.C. Keynote speaker, First Lady Barbara Bush, 1989.

Mother and the late Jill Ireland at the Komen Awards Luncheon, 1987.

Former First Ladies Betty Ford, Nancy Reagan, and Lady Bird Johnson at the Komen Awards Luncheon, 1988.

Former Vice President and Mrs. Quayle preparing for the Washington, D.C., Susan G. Komen "Race for the Cure," June 1990. The proceeds of these nationally held races benefit breast cancer research.

Presenting the President's Cancer Panel subcommittee report on breast cancer to First Lady Hillary Rodham Clinton. Left to right: Donna Shalala, Dr. Jay Harris, Nancy, Mrs. Clinton, and Dr. Harold P. Freeman (1993). *(Photo courtesy of The White House)*

Nancy addressing the United Way in Florida (1993).

Nancy speaking at Minority Breast Cancer Awareness Day (1994).

With Barbara Hawkins of American Airlines at the 1994 Minority Breast Cancer
Awareness Day, Washington D.C. (1994).

With Annie Pearl
Foster, twenty-
year breast cancer
survivor (1994).
*(Photo by Sylvia R.
Dunnavant)*

permanent breast centers. Every day we do our best to reach new women and enlist more fighters in this war.

For information about screening facilities in your area, call the: **Komen Foundation National Tollfree Breast Care Helpline** at 1-800 I'M AWARE (1-800-462-9273) or the **National Cancer Institute** at 1-800 4 CANCER.

To this day, I am saddened by the untimely death of my sister. But I am with her every day through the Susan G. Komen Breast Cancer Foundation. The gift she gave me in life is one that I will cherish always, but the gift she gave me in death is the one for which I will be eternally grateful. It is also the gift she gives the world. If Suzy hadn't died of breast cancer, the Susan G. Komen Breast Cancer Foundation might never have been born. It would not have become the nation's largest private funder of reasearch dedicated solely to breast cancer, and I would not have been inspired to learn the facts that saved my life or carry out her wish to educate other women.

Now, let's talk about you...

PART TWO

You

Chapter Three

Understanding
Your Breasts

Talking about breasts can be uncomfortable for a lot of people. Unless they are the subject of someone's joke, breasts don't usually come up in cocktail-party conversation. At least that is how it used to be. Our friends who have fought fearlessly to bring AIDS to the forefront of American minds have made breast cancer much easier to talk about in comparison. Breast cancer is not contagious, and that is probably why there is little feeling of urgency about the disease. Unlike AIDS, you can't get breast cancer from having sex or through blood transfusions. But it does threaten a woman's sexuality by virtue of its effect on her self-image. It also threatens her life.

A young girl's first sign that she is entering puberty usually comes when her breasts begin to develop. As she privately watches herself begin to grow, secret dreams of entering womanhood take shape. Developing breasts is a sure sign of more exciting things to come, though at that age she is still unclear as to what it all means. At first the impact her breasts will have on the young boys is far less important than the impact they will

> *I'm just a person trapped inside a woman's body.*
>
> ELAYNE BOOSLER

have on the other young girls. *Whose breasts are bigger? Who will get the first bra?*

Eventually, through school-yard talk, motion pictures, television, and books, we start to become aware of the effect our breasts have on boys. As puberty turns into the teen-age years, we do what we can to make them look larger because we are taught to believe this makes us more appealing.

For Suzy, who grew up in the era when Marilyn Monroe was the big screen idol, having a curvaceous figure was very important. Tight sweaters were all the rage back then and she was very much aware that her good looks were credited to more than just a pretty face. Although there was only a three-year difference in our ages, Suzy and I were on the tail end of two entirely different eras as far as what style was in vogue when we entered our adult lives. While my sister and her friends were striving for a look of voluptuous femininity, my friends and I believed that "thin was in." Twiggy was our idol, and we strived for a look of slender elegance. For Suzy and me, the timing of the fashion trends was ideal. She was shorter than I am, about five feet, five inches, and although she was never overweight, her figure was just like an hourglass. By the time I reached college, my height had caught up to my body weight and at almost six feet, I was tall and thin (the thin part was and continues to be a struggle). Our perceptions on what measurements constituted the perfect female figure were based on current fashion trends, peer input, and particular body types, and so differed dramatically. But, regardless of the differences, our individual self-images were extremely important and personal to us.

The importance of a woman's breasts to her total sexuality is embedded deeply in her mind at a very tender age. This happens long before a young girl can even begin to fathom the real physiological purpose of her breasts, which is, of course, to feed her babies. Although her maternal instincts are often nurtured in childhood through the use of dolls, those dolls come with a pretend bottle to complete the fantasy. Today, with the current trend toward natural childbirth and child care, it is likely that a young girl will have the opportunity to watch her mother breastfeed a younger sibling. But, when Suzy and I were growing up, most children were bottle-fed; consequently, many women of our generation never fully understood that breasts were more than sexual objects. I know I didn't.

Even during the now commonplace *sex education* courses in the classroom, more time was spent on intercourse and pregnancy prevention than on breasts. Many teen-agers, although finding it fun to say they are taking sex education, are still embarrassed by the subject and are reluctant to ask questions in front of their peers.

The point is that it is not uncommon for a woman to enter adulthood having little more knowledge about her breasts than the best way to display them in a dress. In order for any of us to truly understand breast cancer, we must first understand the basic anatomy of the breasts, and how they function. Moreover, if we understand how our breasts function normally, we will be able to notice things that are not normal that might be signs of trouble. Too often, women wait until they feel pain before they go to their doctors. With breast cancer, this can be too late, for in its early stages it usually causes no pain. We need to take charge of our own health by understanding our bodies and not relying solely on our doctors to take care of us.

The Anatomy and Physiology of the Breasts

Each woman's breasts are unique in size and shape. The differences are based on one's heredity and total body weight.

Cosmetic plastic surgery must also be considered a variable today because of its growing popularity. Many women have breast enlargements to make them feel more feminine and attractive, while others try to improve their self-image by having breast reductions.

Breasts are glandular organs physiologically designed for one particular purpose: to produce milk. The structure of a woman's breasts changes dramatically throughout her lifetime, especially during the years between puberty and menopause. The normal cycle of female hormones affects both the outward appearance and the inside structure of the breasts, making visible changes almost daily. By understanding these normal changes as they occur, you will be better able to recognize any unusual changes that serve as warning signals for potential problems. But even if you *never* have a problem, it is important to know what is happening to your body. It is no longer acceptable for women to merely go along for the ride where their health is concerned. We have to drive the car. We have been content, in the past, to turn our bodies over to our doctors unconditionally as soon as *they* point out the first sign of trouble. Many people never see a doctor or a dentist unless they feel a pain. But this is a new era in health care. With routine checkups, problems can be identified early when they are most easily treated. By knowing how our bodies are supposed to be functioning, we can use the medical profession to support our wellness rather than merely to treat our sickness.

It is crucial for a woman to understand the physiology of her breasts as well as their anatomical structure because of the close proximity of the breasts to other vital organs such as the heart, lungs, and liver. (Although a man's breasts are located in the same place, their mass, weight, and function do not have the same impact on the body.) The outward appearance of the breasts varies from woman to woman. Obviously, the size of the breasts might vary but there are other common differences as well. Nipples might vary in color and appearance as might the areola. Some women might have small hairs and/or bumps around the areola, others might be smooth and clear. These differences are nothing to worry about.

If you could look underneath the skin and see how the breast is structured, it would look very much like the diagram on page 78. There are five major parts to the female breast; the lymph nodes, the fibrous tissue, the mammary glands and ductal system, the fat tissue, and the nipple and areola.

- *THE LYMPH NODES*: soft, bean-shaped structures which are the filtering devices of a microscopic network of tiny channels known as the lymphatic system that drain body tissue fluids and carry fluids that help the body fight infection. Fluids from the breasts drain primarily to lymph node chains located under the arm. The underarm or axillary lymph nodes become quite important in breast cancer because they are one of the first regions to which the cancer can spread.

- *THE FIBROUS TISSUE*: extends from just beneath the surface of the skin to the chest wall muscles to provide support for the breast. It also separates the breast into segments. Younger women have much more fibrous tissue, allowing for firmer breasts.

- *THE MAMMARY GLANDS AND DUCTAL SYSTEM*: The mammary glands are the milk-producing glands. During pregnancy milk is produced in the fifteen to twenty separate lobes of the glands and carried through ducts to the nipples during breast-feeding. The ductal system drains milk from the mammary glands to the nipple.

- *THE FAT TISSUE*: forms a covering for the breast. Its amount varies according to a woman's weight and age. After menopause, the mammary glands begin to shrink and are replaced by fat, causing the breasts to lose their firmness.

- *THE NIPPLE AND AREOLA*: The nipple sticks out from the breast. The ducts that carry milk from the mammary glands lead to the nipple, from which the milk is drawn by a nursing baby. The areola is the dark area of skin surrounding the nipple.
- *THE CHEST WALL*: consists of the ribs and a large group of muscles that fan out over them. These muscles and ribs form the firm background to which the breast is attached.

Normal Hormonal Changes in the Breasts

The breasts change in reaction to the cyclic fluctuation of the female hormones, both estrogen and progesterone, throughout a woman's lifetime. Some cyclic changes women experience include subtle enlargement and shrinkage of the breasts as we near and end our menstrual cycle and pain that comes and goes monthly. There is the natural re-shaping of the breasts that comes with age, childbirth, and weight loss or gain. During puberty, estrogen production begins and affects the growth of the mammary glands. Fat in the breast increases and fibrous tissue becomes more elastic. Complete development of the breast occurs after ovulation begins with the effect of progesterone on the mammary glands. Just prior to menstruation the breasts are particularly tender.

During the menstrual cycle, changes in size and firmness take place because of changes in hormone balance. Breasts become larger, firmer, and more tender just before menstruation in preparation for a possible pregnancy. There is fluid retention and swelling of the duct glands. All areas of the breast are not affected to the same degree. Certain areas might be more tender or painful than others. As the cycle continues and pregnancy does not occur, the breasts readjust themselves. The swelling goes down and the tenderness subsides. When there is a pregnancy, the changes in the breast become more extreme due to the swelling and growth of the mammary glands and ducts. Breast-feeding maintains milk production in these glands. During menopause, the breasts become smaller and softer because of the shrinking of mammary glands. At this time, the mammary glands are replaced with fat.

Becoming familiar and comfortable with these changes will help you to understand what your breasts are supposed to look and feel like on a normal basis. It will also become an invaluable piece of knowledge on which to base your concerns should you see or feel something that is *not* normal for you.

But how do you know what is or isn't normal for you? By examining your breasts routinely each month through a regular process known as breast self-examination. This process is described below. Your doctor should also chart what is normal for you by conducting an annual clinical breast exam and by ordering a screening mammogram (X ray examination of the breast).

Detecting Changes That Are Not Normal

The same three processes that indicate what is normal for your breasts—breast self-examination, clinical breast exam, and screening mammography—are also the best possible tools for finding problems in your breasts. Before discussing these tools, however, I should point out that not all breast abnormalities are cancerous. Hundreds of thousands of women experience breast lumps or other abnormalities at some time in their lives and never have cancer. So if an abnormality appears, you need not panic.

Breast Self-Examination

Breast self-examination (BSE) is one of the finest health habits a woman can acquire. Developing this habit is one way of taking charge of your body and becoming a responsible custodian of your own good health. A breast self-exam is an uncomplicated three-step process, requiring only a few minutes of your time each month. The best time to examine your breasts is just as your period is ending, or for postmenopausal women, the same day of each month. Pregnant women should examine their breasts the same day of each month, as should breast-feeding mothers. Nursing mothers should feed babies just before breast self-examination.

The key to the success of BSE is to practice the process religiously every single month. Remember, you will be looking and feeling for *changes* in how your breasts normally look or feel. Skipping a month or two can make an enormous difference in accuracy of the exam. After you have done BSE a few times, you will become familiar with the contour of your breasts, and a problem, should one arise, will be something you can sense instinctively as well as feel.

The first part of BSE is visual, looking for changes from *your* normal; the second and third parts are palpation, feeling for changes from your normal.

Step One:

Performed in front of a mirror and in good light. Visually examine your breasts in the following positions, remembering to look from the collarbone to the base of the breast and from the breastbone to the underarm area:

   A. *With arms at side:* Simply look at your breasts. They are not usually exactly alike. Check for lumps, thickenings, dimples, or differences in skin color, all of which could be signs of a problem.

B. *With arms over head:* Look for any changes from the normal appearance of your breasts.

C. *With your hands on your hips:* Press down on your hip bone. This will tense your chest muscles. Look for any changes from normal.

D. Finally, check for changes in the appearance of the nipple. Squeeze each nipple very gently and check for discharge; either a discharge when none was previously present or a change in color or amount.

Step Two:

Performed lying down on your back. This position helps to spread the breast across the chest, making examination easier.

A. Place a pillow under your right shoulder and put your right arm behind your head. With fingers flat, use your left hand to press gently against the breast using one of these three methods:

- *(Circular)* Beginning at the outer edge, press the flat part of your fingers in small circles, moving the circles slowly around the entire breast from the collarbone to below the breast, including the underarm area. Gently squeeze nipple to check for discharge.

- *(Vertical)* Move your fingers up and down the breast in a line, beginning from the collarbone and working toward the nipple, then from the nipple continuing to below the breast. Include the underarm area. Gently squeeze nipple to check for discharge.

- *(Wedge)* Divide your breast into imaginary wedges and move your fingers away from the nipple to the outer edge of the breast, then back toward the nipple in each wedge. Remember, the breast area is from the collarbone to the bottom of the breast and includes the underarm area. Gently squeeze nipple to check for discharge.

B. Repeat for left breast.

Step Three:

Performed while bathing.

A. Raise your right arm straight up behind your head. With your left hand soaped and fingers held flat together, press your right breast firmly against the chest wall. Using the circular motion in step two, check for any lumps or thickenings as you did in step two.

B. Repeat this process with the left breast.

Once you become comfortable with this simple procedure, it should only take you about five or ten minutes each month. If you notice any irregularities or if anything seems even the slightest bit different to you from the previous month, do not hesitate to call your physician. Don't panic, but do see your health-care professional.

If for any reason—physical or psychological—you have difficulty doing a monthly breast self-examination, find a good nurse practitioner and have that person examine your breasts at least once every three months.

Clinical Breast Exam

In conjunction with your mammogram and breast self-exam, it is important to have a regular breast exam given by your doctor. A small percentage of breast lumps are not detected by mammography, but can be felt during a clinical breast examination. Therefore, it is very important that women have *both* a clinical breast examination and a screening mammogram performed. A physician who has been trained in breast examination is sensitive to abnormalities you and I might miss on our own, especially if we have been negligent in performing our breast self-examinations. Many women have their breasts examined by their gynecologists, others by their family doctor. Ask your doctor if he or she gives the exam regularly. If the answer is no, ask to be referred to someone who is knowledgeable in the practice.

The exam will consist of essentially the same procedure described in BSE. It should include a visual exam and palpation while sitting and lying down.

Mammography

Perhaps the best line of defense against breast cancer is mammography. A mammogram is an X ray of the breast. Many women resist having a mammogram because they fear exposure to radiation. When mammography was first developed, this fear might have had some substance because the dosage ranged from six to eight rads per view, but today this fear is totally unfounded because new low-dose techniques have been developed that are not dangerous and do not cause cancer. Low-dose mammography is widely available now and can obtain fine-quality results while exposing women to less than one rad per mammogram, which is less than a dental X ray.

Low-dose mammography can detect tumors as small in size as a few grains of salt. Do you realize that the survival rate is 95 percent when tumors are discovered that small? For a tumor to be felt, or palpated, by even the most trained human hand, it would have to be at least the size of a pea. Many tumors are larger than this when first found, and most probably have been growing inside the body for several years or longer. When a cancerous tumor has been allowed to grow for that long, the chances are far greater that an aggressive cancer will have spread or metastasized outside the confines of the breast. The

Breast self-exam.

Courtesy of the Susan G. Komen Breast Cancer Foundation
**For more information call 1-800-I'm Aware.
(1-800-462-9273)**

Check Your Breast Using These Steps:

1

Lying down: Place a pillow under your right shoulder. Put your right hand under your head. Check your entire breast area with the finger pads of your left hand. Use small circles and follow an up and down pattern. Use light, medium and firm pressure over each area of your breast. Gently squeeze the nipple for any discharge. Repeat these steps on your left breast.

2

Before a mirror: Check for any changes in the shape or look of your breasts. Note any skin or nipple changes such as dimpling or nipple discharge. In-spect your breasts in four steps: arms at side, arms overhead, hands on hips pressing firmly to flex chest muscles, and bending forward.

3

In the shower: Raise your right arm. With soapy hands and fingers flat, check your right breast. Use the method described in the "Lying Down" step. Repeat on your left breast.

The Komen Foundation and the American Cancer Society urge women to consider the following:

WHAT YOU SHOULD DO IF YOU FIND A CHANGE
If you find a lump or dimple or discharge during BSE, it is important to see your doctor as soon as possible. Don't be frightened. Most breast lumps or changes are not cancer, but only your doctor can make the diagnosis.

WHY YOU SHOULD EXAMINE YOUR BREASTS MONTHLY
Most breast cancers are first discovered by women themselves. Since breast cancers found early and treated promptly have excellent chances for cure, learning how to examine your breasts properly can help save your life. Use the simple three-step breast self-examination (BSE) procedure shown here. Remember, you are not necessarily looking for cancer. Eighty-percent of all breast lumps are benign. What you need to learn to do is carefully "read" your breast tissue with your fingers for changes that only you may be able to detect.

FOR THE BEST TIME TO EXAMINE YOUR BREASTS:
Follow the same procedure once a month about a week after the start of your period, when breasts are usually not tender or swollen. After menopause, check breasts on the first day of each month. After hysterectomy, check with your doctor or clinic for an appropriate time of the month. Doing BSE will give you monthly peace of mind. Every woman should have a regular checkup with a breast examination.

fact is that the survival rate for women whose breast cancer has been detected early by mammography is between 90 and 95 percent, while the survival rate for women whose cancer has been detected by palpation is much less, because cancers detected by mammography are often at a much earlier stage of their development.

Dr. G. W. Eklund, who heads the Komen Breast Center in Peoria, Illinois, explains the situation as clearly as anyone I've ever heard. "There are yet no known methods or devices to prevent breast cancer. The terrible realization that during her lifetime one of every nine women in the United States will develop breast cancer is made even worse by the reality that the incidence is increasing. The mortality rate remains the same as it has for decades (more than forty-five thousand deaths annually). In spite of it all, there is good news, even better news, and some of the best of all news. The good news is, there is a kind of breast cancer that is curable! The even better news is, almost all breast cancers are, at some stage in their development, this kind of curable cancer! The best of all news is, we have the ability to find these curable breast cancers! *Curable breast cancer is early cancer!*"

Knowing that mammography is currently the best way to detect early breast cancer, it is nothing less than horrifying to learn that still only 34 percent of all women over the age of fifty follow the recommendations for a yearly screening mammogram. Yet, most women over the age of eighteen *have* had a gynecological exam. Why do you suppose a woman would be so conscientious about the health of one part of her body and so negligent about the health of another? The answer is probably fear. Fear of hearing something she doesn't want to hear. Fear of losing a breast. Fear of abandonment by a loved one. And fear of losing her life.

But there is no need to be afraid. You should know that 80 percent of all breast abnormalities are not cancerous. Moreover, if the 20 percent of breast lumps that are cancerous are detected in their earliest stages, the likelihood of losing a breast is dramatically decreased. More important, the likelihood of death from breast cancer is also dramatically decreased.

Another reason women are reluctant to get a mammogram is the expense. It can cost up to two hundred fifty dollars for a mammogram. The Komen Foundation and the National Cancer Institute together with other organizations have been successful in convincing legislatures in some states to change their laws so that screening mammography is covered by insurance for women thirty-five years of age and older. This has been a major advance in the war against breast cancer. It is important that you know and understand exactly what the laws are in your own state regarding mammography. But even if mammography is not covered by your insurance, think carefully about its value and the relatively low cost in comparison to your own good health and peace of mind.

Congress passed the Breast and Cervical Cancer Mortality Prevention Act in 1990. Through this act programs have been and continue to be established offering breast and cervical education and screening with emphasis on the older, low-income, underinsured, and uninsured woman.

WHO SHOULD HAVE A MAMMOGRAM?

Although the National Cancer Institute recently changed its recommendations for screening mammography in women aged forty to forty-nine, more than *twenty* other organizations still recommend screening mammography in this age group. The controversy concerning mammography in this age group centers on whether screening improves survival. In clinical trials that were reviewed by the NCI in which no statistical survival benefits were noted, the number of patients in the forty to forty-nine age group were under-represented and follow-up was too short. The NCI has been asked to review its present change in recommendations at a consensus conference.

"It is important to know that approximately 35 percent of breast cancers in this age group are detected by mammography alone. It is also felt by many clinicians that screening in this age group increases the potential for breast conservation. Most clinicians therefore continue to recommend screening in this age group until future randomized studies can better clarify the data or until better modalities for detection are developed," says Dr. George Peters, a surgical oncologist.

The Komen Foundation and the American Cancer Society agree that every woman should begin screening mammography by age forty. (A screening mammogram is an X ray taken in an asymptomatic woman to detect any abnormality that might indicate early signs of breast cancer.) A woman under forty with either a family history of breast cancer or other concerns about her risk should consult with her physician about when to begin screening mammograms. A mammogram every one to two years is recommended for women ages forty to forty-nine. Because over 75 percent of all breast cancers occur in women over fifty, yearly mammograms are recommended thereafter for screening purposes.

If your physician does not suggest a mammogram for you, suggest one for yourself. By now you understand the immeasurable importance of the mammogram and its value in your future. Be the custodian of your own good health. If at all possible, try to have your mammogram performed at the same medical office and/or by the same clinician each year to make the comparison easier. Your X rays will be stored in the facility where your mammogram is done. If you decide to change doctors and/or facilities, ask to have your X rays forwarded to the new physician and/or location.

If you or your physician notice any change in how your breasts normally look or feel, you may be referred for a diagnostic mammogram. (A diagnostic mammogram is an X ray taken to further evaluate an already palpable lump or some other abnormality or an abnormal screening mammogram.) Remember that my sister's breast cancer was detected at the age of thirty-three and she died at thirty-six.

Screening Guidelines

as recommended by The Komen Foundation and the American Cancer Society.

• Beginning by age 40
• Age 40-49—screening mammogram every one to two years
• Age 50 and over—screening mammogram annually

WHAT IS INVOLVED IN A MAMMOGRAM?

The procedure is quite simple, takes only a few minutes, and is relatively painless. I say relatively painless because there can be a few minutes of slight discomfort involved. A typical mammogram consists of two views of each breast, top to bottom and side to side. In order to obtain the most accurate picture, the breast is pressed firmly between two plates. For women with especially sensitive breasts, this can feel a bit uncomfortable, though most women feel no discomfort whatsoever. Premenopausal women can minimize pain by having their mammogram done between five and seven days after their period ends. If you are feeling too much discomfort, tell your technician. Think of it this way: It is less painful, has to be done a lot less often, and does you much more good than tweezing your eyebrows.

GUIDELINES FOR GETTING THE BEST POSSIBLE
MAMMOGRAM FOR YOUR TIME AND MONEY
In 1992, Congress passed the Mammography Quality Standards
Act (MQSA) to ensure that all mammography done at the
approximately eleven thousand facilities in this country is safe
and reliable. The Food and Drug Administration has the responsibility for implementing and enforcing the MQSA.

By October 1, 1994, mammography facilities in the United
States must meet quality standards established by the FDA or
cease operation. The new standards require:

- that X ray images be of high quality; that the personnel
  who perform mammography and the physicians who
  interpret the mammography have adequate training and
  experience;
- that mammography facilities be inspected annually by
  FDA-trained inspectors;
- that mammography units be monitored closely to ensure
  radiation levels and overall operation;
- that mammography facilities set up quality assurance programs to ensure that mammograms are as clear as possible.

The FDA has issued certificates to certified mammography facilities which should be prominently displayed so that women will
know the facility is certified and has met the required standards.
Facilities that have applied for, but not yet received, accreditation have been issued a provisional certificate, valid for six
months, allowing them to legally provide mammography services while their application is being reviewed.

For a listing of accredited facilities in your area, call The
Susan G. Komen Breast Cancer Foundation National Tollfree
Breast Care Helpline at 1-800 I'M AWARE (1-800-462-9273), the

American College of Radiology (ACR 1-800-227-6440), or the Cancer Information Service (CIS) at 1-800 4 CANCER.

In summary, I cannot stress enough the importance of a mammogram. Detecting cancer early is your absolute best defense against advanced breast cancer.

Susan Blumenthal, M.D., M.P.A., deputy assistant secretary for health (Women's Health) and assistant attorney general in the United States Department of Health and Human Services, has launched an exciting new initiative to improve the early detection of breast cancer. She comments, "It seems logical that if our military science and technology can image missiles 15,000 miles away and with the Hubble telescope see the surface of Mars, we should be able to develop better tools to image small tumors in women's breasts that are right in front of us!" To that end, she has initiated a collaboration between the Public Health Service's Office on Women's Health and the National Cancer Institute to explore the application of methods from the defense, space, intelligence and computer graphics fields (that are estimated to be ten years ahead of medical imaging capacities) to improve the early detection of breast cancer.

The translation of imaging technologies from defense to breast cancer detection is imminently feasible, and the collaborations have begun from *missiles to mammograms.* "This nation can realize no greater peace dividend from our national investment in defense than to save the lives of American women," states Dr. Blumenthal.

Benign Breast Disease

Noticing something abnormal in the breast will cause an intelligent woman some concern—it ought to. But as I pointed out

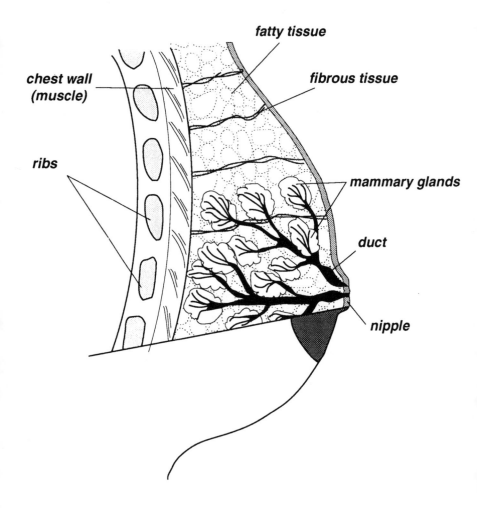

Diagram of a Healthy Breast

earlier, it need not provoke immediate fright or panic. Eighty percent of all breast lumps are benign, which means noncancerous.
There are many benign breast conditions that mimic cancer and
can frighten many women unnecessarily. Brief descriptions of
the most common of these conditions follow. Becoming knowledgeable about them should help you to understand more about
your body and how it works, and make you feel more at ease if
you notice anything unusual in your breasts. The important thing
is to react immediately if you do notice anything. If you are even
a little bit suspicious about anything at all, have it checked right
away by a respected health-care professional. Worrying is a waste
of your time. The odds are that you don't have breast cancer, but
if you do—waiting will only make it worse.

*Please note: These descriptions must not be used to self-
diagnose. If you have a lump of any sort, see your doctor.*

Fibrocystic Breast Changes

This non-threatening condition, in which multiple tiny cysts
develop in one or, usually, both breasts, is by far the most common benign breast condition. The breasts might have an overall
lumpy feel or distinct lumpy areas, which might be accompanied by tenderness or discomfort that fluctuates with the menstrual cycle, increasing just before the period begins. The
condition, which is also referred to by doctors as mammary dys-
plasia or chronic cystic mastitis, is generally thought to be the
breasts' response to hormonal levels as they change from month
to month over the years. Many types of treatments are recommended to alleviate these symptoms, including milk analgesics,
warm compresses or sleeping bras, a low-salt diet, restriction of
caffeine (coffee, tea, colas, and chocolate), vitamin E supplements, and for the most severe cases, a special type of hormone
treatment. Sometimes, individual cysts or distinct lumps might

be felt. In this case, doctors usually perform a needle aspiration to evaluate the cause (see pages 88-89 for a description of this procedure).

Now I need to say something *very* important. Please don't let the fact that both Suzy and I had fibrocystic disease *and* cancer frighten you unduly. This, as far as we know, was just a coincidence. If you have lumpy breasts, it does not mean you are more likely to develop cancer. It does mean that you need to be especially aware of the normal changes your breasts go through regularly so that your hand and eye are alert to changes that might be abnormal. With that in mind, remember that *nearly all women's breasts develop some degree of lumpiness.*

Fibroadenoma

Fibroadenoma is a solid benign tumor composed of fibrous and glandular tissue. It is painless and movable and has a rubbery feel. Usually it occurs singularly, but occasionally multiple fibroadenoma can occur. Although this tumor is most frequently found in women ages twenty to forty, fibroadenomas are the most common mass found in girls prior to puberty.

Cysts

Cysts are fluid-filled sacs. In the breast, they can be small enough to go unnoticed by the hand and eye or large enough to hold as much as a quarter cup of fluid. You could have one or two isolated cysts, or fibrocystic disease, which is recurring cysts.

Ductal Papillomas

Ductal papillomas are small, benign, finger-like growths in the mammary ducts close to the nipple. The growths, which are usually difficult to feel, cause a bloody discharge from the nipple.

This condition occurs most often in, but is not limited to, women between the ages of forty-five and fifty.

Mammary Duct Ectasia

This is a condition unique to women near or past menopause, wherein the ducts behind the nipples become enlarged and inflamed. A lump might or might not be present. Symptoms are burning and itching around the nipple or occasionally a dark discharge from the nipple.

Fat Necrosis

Fat necrosis, the death of tissue following an injury or surgery to the breast, usually results in a painful lump. This condition can occur at any age.

Galactocele

This is a clogged milk duct associated with childbirth that can affect both breast-feeding and non-breast-feeding mothers.

In Summary

Although an abnormality in your breasts does not necessarily mean cancer, this does not mean you can ignore it or put off consulting your doctor about it. It is important to have a diagnosis made as soon as possible so that if it should be cancer, you can catch it before it has a chance to spread.

In the next chapter I describe what should be done if an abnormality appears, and how a diagnosis is made.

CHAPTER FOUR

Understanding Breast Cancer and How It Is Diagnosed

I f an abnormality should appear in one of your breasts, you will need to discover as soon as possible whether it is a benign breast disease or cancer. In order to understand what needs to be done, it is important that you know something about breast cancer itself.

Life is something that happens to you while you're making other plans.

MARGARET MILLAR

Understanding breast cancer won't enable you to escape the disease, but it could save your life. It saved mine. At present there is nothing we can do to prevent breast cancer. There is some work being done to show how a low-fat diet might be beneficial. But if we catch it in its earliest stage, optimally we can expect a 95-percent chance of survival. To me, that makes it worth learning about.

What Is Breast Cancer?

The words "breast cancer" strike fear in the hearts of everyone, and some people won't talk about it. The truth is, no one likes to talk about cancer. And because no one likes to talk about it, many people don't even know what it is, other than a disease that can kill you. I will try to define it here in simple terms.

Healthy cells that make up the body's tissue grow, divide, and replace themselves in an orderly manner. Sometimes cells lose their ability to control their growth. They divide too rapidly and grow out of control, forming masses or tumors. These tumors, which can expand by invading and destroying healthy tissues and organs, are cancer. Cancerous tumors are called malignant because they are potentially fatal. Tumors can also arise in the body that do not spread by invasion and are therefore not usually life-threatening. These noncancerous tumors are referred to as benign. (An example of a benign tumor is the fibroadenoma, discussed on page 80.) A malignant tumor is very dangerous because it can invade healthy tissues and organs not only locally (adjacent to itself) but also in other parts of the body, to which it travels through the bloodstream and the lymphatic system. This systemic spreading, known as metastasis, usually does not occur until the cancer has grown for a period of time.

Some breast cancers remain confined to either the duct or lobule (in situ cancer), while others grow into the surrounding tissue (invasive or infiltrating). The most common type of breast cancer is infiltrating ductal carcinoma. Breast cancer can spread regionally to the underarm or axillary lymph nodes. Spread to distant body areas is referred to as metastasis. The most common areas for metastasis are the lungs, bones, liver, and brain.

Signs of Breast Cancer

When breast cancer begins, it rarely causes pain or other obvious symptoms that might alert you that something is wrong. But as a cancerous growth develops, it might take on several different outward appearances that act as warning signs.

- *A LUMP*: most often felt and not seen by the human eye in

its early stages. It is usually single, hard, and painless.
- *NIPPLE CHANGE*: Every once in a while, a nipple will be naturally inverted. But if you notice your nipple becoming inverted after previously being normal, this could be a sign of danger.
- *SKIN SWELLING*: when a portion of the skin becomes red and swollen, much like the appearance of an orange peel.
- *SUPERFICIAL VEINS*: when the veins closest to the skin become obviously more prominent on one breast than the other.
- *SKIN DIMPLING*: when a depression occurs in a particular area of the breast surface.

These are the most obvious warning signals for breast cancer. However, it cannot be stressed enough that if you notice anything at all out of the ordinary, you should report it to your doctor immediately.

If an Abnormality Appears

Let's go over exactly what should be done, step by step, in the event of even the most minute abnormality. I like to use plain language, for I know how intimidating medical terminology can be. If you thoroughly understand it now, you will be better able to recall the information at the time when you need it most. Keep in mind that no two cases of breast cancer are exactly the same. Diagnosis and treatment procedures must be individualized according to many factors unique to the woman involved. However, it is useful to understand what the various possibilities are so that, if nothing else, you have a starting point on which to base your own questions.

Signs of breast disorder.

Inverted nipple.

Skin swelling. Note the swollen area
around the nipple.

Inflammatory carcinoma, characterized
by a rash-like area.

Photos courtesy of Dr. George Peters

The First Step: Finding the Right Doctor

If you have a lump in your breast, chances are that it was detected one of four ways: (1) You found it yourself through BSE or by accident (which was the way I found my own cancer); (2) it was noticed by a sexual partner and brought to your attention; (3) it was discovered by your doctor during a medical exam; or (4) it showed up during a screening mammogram. If the lump was detected by options 3 or 4, your advantage is that at least you are under a doctor's supervision. You have a place to begin, someone to whom you can direct your questions. But if you found the lump yourself or if it was found by a sexual partner, where do you go first? Whom do you call?

Women in the United States most often turn to their gynecologists when they have any kind of personal physical problem. For this reason, many GYNs have made it a point to become knowledgeable about breast diseases. Whether you choose to see your gynecologist, a general practitioner, or any other family doctor you feel comfortable with, don't hesitate for a moment to ask if he or she has a special interest in the detection and diagnosis of breast disease. If the answer is no, ask to be referred to a breast specialist. Even if the answer is yes, you might want to see a breast specialist for evaluation, confirmation, and additional tests if they become necessary.

You should be aware that a breast specialist is a rather rare commodity. "It is sad," admits Dr. G. W. Eklund, head of the Komen Breast Center in Peoria, Illinois, "that so many physicians providing primary care for women openly admit their omission of a breast examination as part of the routine physical, or frankly admit that they feel poorly equipped to evaluate and treat breast disorders, benign or malignant. Considering the magnitude of breast-related diseases, it is curious if not tragic that the study of the breast has not emerged as a major field of practice. We are beginning to see more surgeons taking an additional fellowship year in breast surgery and limiting their practice to diseases of the breast. Radiologists are doing the same thing with regard to diagnostic imaging of the breast."

But what if you are without a physician at all? Perhaps you are new to an area or on vacation. Usually everyone has access to a nearby hospital that can refer them to a specialist. In the event you are in an extremely rural part of the country or are not comfortable with the physician you know, there are several organizations listed in the Resource section of this book that can help you find a good physician, cancer specialist, hospital, or clinic as nearby as possible.

Diagnostic Testing

Once a lump is detected and you are in the care of a doctor you trust, there are several important diagnostic steps that can follow. First, if you haven't had a *mammogram*, you will. This will give both you and your doctor a clearer picture of the specific location of the lump and its exact size.

It is possible your lump might be nothing more than a fluid-filled cyst. If this is the case, it can be determined immediately, in the doctor's office by a "*needle aspiration*." Using a needle and syringe, your doctor will attempt to extract fluid from the lump. If you have a cyst, the syringe will fill up with fluid and the wall of the cyst will collapse, much like what would happen if you poked a needle into a balloon filled with water.

If the lump is solid, nothing will be obtained by aspiration and a *biopsy* will be in order. A biopsy might also be in order if the fluid extracted from the cyst is bloody or looks suspicious in any way. Biopsy, the removal and microscopic examination of tissue to see if cancer cells are present, is discussed on page 89.

There are other tests that might be suggested to get a different perspective on the suspicious mass before a biopsy is performed. It is important that you know what they are and their purpose in order to make the experience less frightening. Remember that none of these tests has been proven effective enough to replace mammography screening. They must be used in conjunction with your mammogram or not at all. A mammogram can more clearly define whether a mass or lump has clear margins—that is, clear edges.

- *ULTRASONOGRAPHY:* uses sound waves to produce echoes which can be photographed and viewed on a screen. These sound waves can distinguish the presence of an abnormal tissue and can separate solid from fluid-filled (cystic) masses. Ultrasound might provide guidance for needle aspiration or fine-needle biopsy of nonpalpable masses.

- *MAGNETIC RESONANCE IMAGING (MRI:)* a new, experimental technique that uses the interaction between magnetism and radio waves to picture the structure of biological tissues. MRI is too costly to replace mammography as a screening procedure. However, it might be useful as a sophisticated diagnostic tool in cases where conventional methods cannot provide a diagnosis.

Biopsy

Effective as it is in detecting early tumors, mammography has not eliminated the need for surgical biopsy when trying to decipher whether or not a breast mass is benign or malignant. There are four types of biopsy procedures, two of which are surgical.

- *FINE-NEEDLE ASPIRATION:* performed in the doctor's office. A fine needle inserted into the suspicious mass and cells are sucked out, placed on a glass slide, and studied under a microscope.

- *CORE-NEEDLE BIOPSY:* uses a special kind of needle that removes a plug of tissue, which is then examined and studied under a microscope. For non-palpable lumps,

either ultrasonography or mammography might be used
to guide the needle. Core biopsies using mammography as
a guide are also referred to as **stereotactic** biopsies.

- *INCISIONAL BIOPSY*: involves an incision made directly
  over the mass and is used for larger masses that are not
  amenable to the excisional biopsy. This procedure might
  be done on any outpatient basis using either local or general anesthesia.

- *EXCISIONAL BIOPSY*: involves removal of all gross evidence of the lump/mass, usually with a rim of normal tissue. This procedure might be done on an outpatient basis.
  Local or general anesthesia might be used. This is the
  "standard" biopsy procedure.

If fine-needle aspiration or core-needle biopsy fails to provide a
definite diagnosis, then you will need a surgical biopsy, most
likely an excisional biopsy. Generally, the biopsy and any definitive surgery for breast cancer are separated by a space of time
ranging anywhere from several days to two or three weeks. The
important issue is that women do not have to go under anesthesia wondering if they will awake with or without their breast.
Although the tendency is to act quickly and get it—the cancer—
out, there is usually not any medical necessity to do so. Women
need time to get as much information as possible in order to
make an informed decision about treatment choices. Get a second opinion. If breast conservation is offered, see not only the
surgeon, but the radiation oncologist. Talk with a medical oncologist.

The biopsy and surgery are most often scheduled as separate
steps. Recent studies have proven that a *short* delay between
biopsy and treatment will not affect the spread of the disease or
decrease the chance of successful treatment. For the surgical
biopsy you will probably go into a hospital on an outpatient

basis. Usually, several days before the scheduled biopsy, you will have some pre-op lab work done. This might include both blood and urine specimens, possibly a chest X ray and an EKG (electrocardiogram). You will also sign a consent form for the surgical biopsy. While you are under anesthesia, your surgeon will remove the tumor and send it to the pathology department for examination under a microscope. As mentioned in chapter 2, a slice of the suspicious tissue will be frozen so that it can be analyzed in a matter of minutes. A final pathology report (permanent section) will be available approximately three working days following the surgery.

You will be discharged from the outpatient surgery area several hours after you return from the operating room. The effects of the biopsy are relatively mild. Your breast might be sore and/or bruised. You might notice a firmness in the biopsied area; this could last a few months. This is just a bruise or scar tissue and is not something you need to worry about.

Several days following the surgery, the surgeon will discuss treatment options available to you, based on the final pathology report.

Tests Performed at the Time of Biopsy

Besides the tissue being examined microscopically by the pathologist, there are a number of other tests that will be performed on the tissue. Before you biopsy, you and your physician should discuss each test he or she intends to perform and why. It is important that you understand everything that is being done to you so that you can become a partner in your treatment.

HORMONE RECEPTOR ASSAY

It is important that hormone receptor assays (tests) are performed at the time of your biopsy, if a malignancy is found. The

hormone receptor assay—one for estrogen and one for progesterone—will determine whether or not your cancer is hormone-
dependent, and whether hormonal therapy will benefit you now
or later in your treatment. (Hormonal therapy is discussed in
chapter 6.) This assay will give the physician very important
clues about which adjuvant treatment might be more effective.
Estrogen-positive or estrogen-rich tumors tend to respond better to hormone drugs. Estrogen-negative tumors tend to be
treated with chemotherapy. The majority of postmenopausal
women have estrogen-positive tumors, while a smaller number
of premenopausal women have estrogen-positive tumors.
Whether you are pre- or postmenopausal and whether the
tumor is estrogen negative or positive will impact the treatment
decision markedly. Any woman with a breast cancer diagnosis
should ask about the results of her hormone receptor tests. Be
aware that it might take as long as seven to ten days to get the
results of these tests back from the laboratory.

FLOW CYTOMETRY
Another test commonly performed today on cancerous tissue at
the time of biopsy is called flow cytometry, which shows the
aggressiveness of the tumor. This test can be performed on the
same tissue as hormone receptors. Flow cytometry yields two
results: whether the cancer has extra chromosomes (aneu-
ploidy) and how fast it is growing (S-phase). Knowing how fast
your cancer is growing is an important factor in determining
your treatment options.

Other Tests That Might Be Performed
CATHEPSIN D
This assay must be performed at the time of the biopsy.
Cathepsin D is an enzyme that is secreted by normal cells but is
produced in greater amounts by breast cancer cells. High levels

of this enzyme increase the risk for recurrence. Once the test becomes more conclusive it might prove to be a very important prognostic indicator.

ONCOGENE TESTING

An oncogene is a genetic defect that causes the cell to go haywire and to multiply at an abnormal speed to produce other abnormal cells. In other words, the oncogene initiates the very first cancerous cell of any cancer that develops. Doctors hope that by developing tests that will reveal the presence of the oncogene in the body, they can take measures to block its effects. The hope is that cancer will be something that can be stopped before it begins. Much research is being done in this area. Soon, physicians will be able to use an assortment of these predictive means to be able to more accurately diagnose a breast cancer, predict recurrence, and prescribe the best treatment.

CHAPTER FIVE

Choosing a Support Team

I f you are diagnosed as having breast cancer, the first thing you must do is try to stay calm. I realize that might seem like a silly thing to say. I didn't stay calm and I was a highly educated cancer patient. But remember this: *Being diagnosed with breast cancer does not mean you have been handed a death sentence.* What it does mean is that you have a serious problem for which you have many options. In the next several chapters I am going to try to guide you through this, as a friend and as a cancer sur-

You have to accept whatever comes and the only important thing is that you meet it with courage and the best you have to give.

ELEANOR ROOSEVELT

vivor. I am not a doctor; I wouldn't presume to give medical advice. What I can do for you, what I want to do for you, is to discuss the disease openly and honestly so that you have a basis for actively participating in the decisions about which options are best for you.

I have found that we, as women, have a tendency to give ourselves up to doctors unconditionally. Dr. Wendy Schain, Director of Adult Psychological Oncology at the Memorial

Cancer Institute, Long Beach, California, once put it this way: "There is something about seeing the two initials M.D. after a name that allows us to give up our right to question their [our doctor's] authority." We must get over this. We owe it to ourselves to ask as many questions as necessary to fully understand our situation.

When you first receive your diagnosis of breast cancer, you will probably be overwhelmed with conflicting emotions.

If there was ever a time for a little self-indulgence, it's now. As Betty Rollin so eloquently put it in her book, *First, You Cry,* you need to allow yourself to release the emotion you feel after being told you have a life-threatening disease. Cry, scream, get mad, feel sorry for yourself—do all of these things if you want. Not only do you deserve it, but expressing yourself honestly will help relieve the stress. But as Betty Ford suggested to me, try to limit the hysteria to a day or two, and then put it behind you. Carrying on indefinitely will affect your ability to take an effective part in the decision-making process now ahead.

It is natural to feel resentful and afraid, victimized and confused. But you need not feel helpless, because there is always something that can be done in an attempt to save or prolong your life. It is your family and those who love you who will feel helpless. You can help them by taking care of yourself.

The best way to take care of yourself I know is to learn as much as you can about what your options are and then decide for yourself which ones best serve your needs—psychologically and practically, as well as medically. To do that you need to assemble a team of experts you trust to give you medical advice and emotional support. Then, ask questions, and keep asking until you understand and are satisfied with the answers. You then will be prepared to embark upon the informed decision-making process that will establish your treatment strategy.

With the help of your team of experts, you can take control of the situation. But remember, the final decisions should be yours.

My Own Support Team

My mother always told me to remember my sense of humor, even in the most difficult situations because those are the times when it is needed most. Whenever I meet a new doctor, whether it is for my own personal health or for the foundation, I can't help but think of Erma Bombeck's funny quote, "Never go to a doctor whose office plants have died."

When cancer was detected in my left breast in 1984, I affectionately referred to the group of people I depended on most during that crucial time period as my "A Team." But the truth is, this group of individuals was and continues to be a guiding force in my life. None of the people on my team were there by accident. I strategized and thought about each one of them and they all have their own individual roles in my continued recovery.

The "A" had a double meaning to me: First, it stood for excellence—representing the best possible group of individuals for my own personal needs; and second, it stood for *attack*. After I got control of my emotions, I was determined to attack my cancer with everything I had.

My advantage over some of you is that my team was pretty much in place *before* my cancer was diagnosed. After living through my sister's illness, going through three previous biopsies, and establishing the Komen Foundation, I already knew which individuals would give me the best possible support I needed, both medically and emotionally. I will share with you how and why the members of my team were chosen, though your needs might be completely different. As in all avenues of cancer treatment, what is right for one person is not necessarily right for another. Every case is different, every woman is an individual. But hearing the way I thought about it might give you a start, if nothing else, in choosing your own A Team. I believe every cancer patient should have one.

The Medical Members

Before I tell you about the medical members of my team, I should mention the various doctors you will need, and why. The best possible team would be a surgeon, an oncologist, a pathologist, a radiologist, and a plastic surgeon. Some programs and centers already have these teams assembled.

The most important factor I used in choosing my medical team was trust. I had to trust my doctors completely, I had to believe wholeheartedly that they wanted to see me well as much as I did. Everything I told my doctors was the truth and I had to believe everything they told me was the truth.

I couldn't have trusted any doctor without being aware of his or her work. Knowing that your oncologist (cancer specialist) is board-certified (approved by the American Medical Association board in his/her subspecialty) should provide an element of comfort. Today, there are over one million new cases of cancer diagnosed yearly in the United States, but only slightly more than five thousand specializing in oncology, or the treatment of cancer. Because of this, cancer patients are naturally being treated by doctors who specialize in other areas. To find out whether or not a physician is board-certified, you can check with the American Medical Association, any of the comprehensive cancer centers, the National Cancer Institute, or the American Society of Clinical Oncology. Or call your county's medical society for a referral. I had the opportunity to interview all my doctors prior to treatment. If you don't have that same advantage, find *one* doctor you trust completely and ask for his or her advice.

I had to like my doctors. This is not to say that I had to become close personal friends with them. If you recall, Suzy felt she had to make her physicians close personal friends, and I have always thought that worked to her disadvantage. Having said that, it just so happened that the person I chose to be my head coach, or team leader, was George Blumenschein, my oncologist. He was and is a good friend and business associate, but that's because we have had the opportunity to develop that kind of a relationship over many years. The doctors you choose to make up your team have got to be willing to spend time with you, particularly the person you choose as your team leader.

If George Blumenschein was my head coach, I was the quarterback. I listened to him and the other members of the team and studied their advice, but I insisted on calling the shots. Of course, I was *capable* of calling the shots, because I was an educated cancer patient. You can be one, too.

I also had two breast surgeons on my team, Fred Ames and George Peters. I was well aware of Fred Ames's work through the time I spent in Houston at M. D. Anderson with Suzy, although she was not his patient. I had interviewed him several times for work with the foundation and knew his work to be first-rate. Fred Ames was the person who performed my mastectomy. George Peters, a breast surgeon in Dallas, where I live, was always willing to answer any question I might have at any time. He was very helpful to me when I labored with lymphedema, guiding me to find a way to overcome the problem rather than just accepting it. Before making these two men a part of my team, I not only interviewed them but I also spoke to some of their patients. (If you need help finding a certified breast surgeon, consult the American College of Surgeons.) Besides the two breast surgeons, I also had two plastic surgeons on the team. Being an informed cancer patient, I knew that down the line, reconstructive surgery would be in my best interest, although I wanted to allow enough time to pass to ensure that I had made a good recovery from my initial surgery. Besides the man who actually performed my surgery in Atlanta, John Bostwick, I depended on (and still depend on) a plastic surgeon in Dallas by the name of Fritz Barton for wise and sound advice. (Considerations involved in breast reconstruction and choosing a reconstructive surgeon are discussed in chapter 7.)

Another medical member on my A Team was Dr. Marc Lippman, an oncologist and the director of the Lombardi Research Center at the Georgetown University Medical Center in Washington, D.C. I have never been a patient of his, but I greatly respect his mind and the contribution he has made to breast cancer research. Dr. Lippman has given me a thoughtful, well-thought-out answer to any question I have ever asked.

And finally, on the medical side of the team was Dr. Stephen Jones, professor of oncology and director of clinical research for the Charles A. Sammons Center at Baylor University Medical Center in Dallas, Texas. He has published extensively in the field of clinical research. He has allowed me to impose on him at any time when I've been confused or unsure. He explains things to me in clear language that I can understand—and repeat, if needed. For this reason, his influence has been immeasurable.

If you think that people of this caliber are unavailable to you, you are mistaken. Ask your primary health-care physician, your local hospital, or the local medical society.

I want to say a word or two about insurance coverage— namely health maintenance organizations (HMOs) and preferred provider organizations (PPOs). This "managed care" has changed the environment when it comes to selecting your physician and your health-care facility. You might not be able to choose your "A Team" like I did. You might be under an HMO or PPO plan. Most physicians are members of some kind of physician network. It is likely that your HMO or PPO will have a wide range of specialists and perfectly good physicians available when you need them.

However, I want you to know that you *do* have some options under this type of "managed care." If your HMO or PPO does not include the specialists needed to treat you, you may negotiate with them so as to seek a physician outside the network. Many HMOs or PPOs are willing to do this. And many physicians outside the network will be willing to see you and accept the fee arrangement set by your HMO or PPO.

If you believe you need to get a second opinion from a physician outside your network, check with your carrier to see if this is a covered expense. Remember, most HMOs or PPOs will work with you to provide the best possible care.

The Emotional Support Members

I believe that to have a winning team, a breast cancer patient needs both medical and emotional support. My requirements for the emotional support team were very much the same as for the medical support team. Each member had to have a great deal of integrity and to be honest with me at all times. I needed empathy without sympathy. I needed people who would not allow me to feel sorry for myself but rather encourage me to continue leading as normal a life as possible. My mother, Ellie Goodman, played a key role in my emotional survival. Without her nurturing every step of the way, I don't know how I would have gotten through the whole ordeal. She never left my side for a moment.

I also received a great deal of strength from talking with other breast cancer patients. There are many women out there who have given me hope and inspiration without even knowing it. *No one* can fully understand exactly what you are going through unless they have been through it themselves. It is important to seek out positive role models if you are going to get strength from other cancer patients. A positive role model is not necessarily a woman who has beaten the disease, but rather a woman who has never given up her will to live. A positive role model has learned to appreciate life *because of* having breast cancer rather than *in spite of* it. In that way, the late Jill Ireland was and will always be a role model for me, as was my dear friend, the late Nina Hyde, fashion editor of *The Washington Post*. Even when their breast cancer was far advanced, both of these women never gave up or gave in. Another was the late Rose Kushner, a former cancer patient and one of the guiding and leading resources in breast cancer research in this country until her death in January 1990. She not only answered my questions but always left me with a provocative thought to ponder long after our conversation ended. Rose Kushner helped me become a stronger cancer survivor.

Another member of my nonmedical support team was my good friend, Sharon McCutchin. Besides being an active member of the Komen Foundation, Sharon is the one person I can *always* count on for a good laugh. Even in my darkest, ugliest moments, she had the ability to cut through my turmoil and bring a smile to my face. I call friends who accept you without makeup and without hair "*low*-maintenance friends"—the best kind to have!

The last two members of my emotional support A Team were my husband, Norman, and son, Eric. Norman is my best friend. He also, without ever trying and perhaps never knowing, inspired me to try to look good throughout my illness. I never wanted him to know how sick I felt, because I didn't want to scare him. Every day I made a conscious effort to fix my hair (or wig, or scarf, or turban) and put on my lipstick so that he would still find me attractive. If I wasn't up to getting dressed, I put on something colorful. Doing these little things made me feel better and if Norman wasn't around, I might not have made the effort. Eric, of course, loves me unconditionally. Until he left for college, not an evening went by without his telling me he loved me. I think that is a lot to get from a son. He, above all else, provided me with the reason to get well, and get well fast.

Your "A Team"

That was my A Team. Once again, what worked for me might not necessarily work for you. Every one of these people was my partner. Those you choose to support you through your illness should have personalities that blend with yours. Your team should consist of the best possible medical advisors you can find, a few people who will love you no matter what you say or do, at least one person who will make you laugh, someone who pushes you to your fullest mental potential, someone who pushes you to your fullest physical potential, and someone for whom you will always want to look pretty. Once your team is set, together you can plan your winning strategy.

A Word on Doctor/Patient Relationships

Gone are the days when we, as women, must accept whatever is said to us without question or confrontation, especially where our health is concerned. As I said at the beginning of this chapter, the best thing you can do for yourself is to ask your doctor as many questions as you need to ask in order to fully understand what has happened, what is happening, and what will happen to your body. Asking questions will also aid in the evolution of good doctor/patient relationships based on understanding and open communication. As the century closes, I see a significant increase in our opportunity to make informed decisions based on our increased education and knowledge. You not only have the right to know the reason for every piece of medical advice you receive, it is now your *responsibility* to know. It is my opinion that once doctors get used to the idea of communicating openly and honestly, they will appreciate sharing the burden of the crucial decisions that must be made daily in dealing with cancer patients. Giving physicians the power to make these critical decisions without the input of their patients might have done wonders for their egos, but it has to have been murder on their stress levels.

The Questioning Process

In developing a successful relationship with your doctor, keep in mind that he or she must be treated with the same respect you insist upon for yourself. Remember that doctors are professionals. Naturally, if you are diagnosed with breast cancer you will have many urgent questions that need to be answered. The best way to handle this, I have found, is to write your questions down and try, as much as possible, to ask all your questions in one sitting. It isn't fair to call your doctor several times a day with questions or to ask for medical advice at a social get-together.

Sometimes a woman can be so preoccupied with the fact that she has cancer that it is nearly impossible for her to remember the answers to the questions she has so painstakingly prepared. This is a normal reaction and one that should not cause any undue embarrassment. What it does call for is a back-up plan. Take notes. Or bring a tape recorder into your doctor's office so you can play the tape containing both your questions and the answers later, at a time when you feel more relaxed and better able to hold onto the information. Another option might be to bring a relative or close friend into the consultation with whom you can discuss the outcome later to make sure you both received the same information.

The important thing is that you *ask* those questions no matter how frightened you are of the answers, no matter how uncomfortable it is to discuss a subject as intimate as your breasts with a virtual stranger.

What questions should you ask? I can give you a guideline, a place to begin. You can and should add to this list whatever else you want to know. No question is silly or stupid when you are fighting for your life.

1. What, specifically, did my biopsy show?
2. What surgical procedures are used to treat breast cancer?
3. What are the potential risks and benefits of these procedures?
4. Which procedure are you recommending for me, and why?
5. Where will the surgical scar or scars be located?
6. How can I expect to look and feel after surgery?
7. Why do doctors take lymph nodes from the armpit area?
8. When will you know about my lymph node involvement?
9. What role does lymph node involvement play in my overall health picture?
10. Is there any indication that my cancer has spread?
11. What were the results of my hormone receptor assays? (Your doctor might not have the results for seven to fourteen days.) What treatment is indicated by those results?
12. What about the aggressiveness of my tumor? How quickly is it growing? What factors helped you to determine this? What does this mean in terms of treatment?

13. Will I need any treatment beyond surgery? Why (or why not)? What supplemental treatments are available?
14. Am I a candidate for breast reconstruction? If so, what options are available to me?
15. If I am a candidate, what steps should be taken to assure successful reconstruction?

These are just a few of the first things you will probably want to know as soon as breast cancer has been diagnosed. After a specific treatment has been suggested, I'm sure you will have a lot more questions. As we discuss the different treatment options in the next chapter, I will add to that list of questions just as you will.

Speaking in Positives

The first question that comes to every woman's mind when she is told she has breast cancer is *Am I going to die?* For many years, cancer and death were two words that went hand in hand. This is not the case anymore. More people are surviving cancer every day. Breast cancer, detected in its earliest stages, has a high percentage of successful outcomes. Asking if you are going to die, though it is an understandable question, is a difficult question for any doctor to answer. It is also very negative and immediately presents an unfavorable state of mind. To put yourself in a more positive state, try to ask questions such as: What can *I* do to beat this? or What can we do as a *team* to ensure my best chances of survival? You have every reason to feel hopeful about getting through this. If you want more constructive answers, ask more constructive questions.

Still, you need to know the facts. No doctor is doing you a favor if he glosses over the seriousness of your condition. But wouldn't you rather think that you have an 85-percent chance of survival than a 15-percent chance of death? Even if I was told I had a 10-percent chance of survival, *that's* what I would hold on to. When you get into the habit of speaking in positives about your condition, it will do wonders for your morale, your relationship with your doctors, and your ability to communicate openly with your family and friends. You will become a positive role model to other cancer patients without ever being conscious of it—perhaps at a time when you might have even considered giving up.

Second Opinions

Once you've prepared your questions, listened to the answers, and discussed them thoroughly, what happens if you are not satisfied with the information you've received? Are you stuck? Let me tell you about my friend Richard Bloch in Kansas City. You might have heard of him, as he is the cofounder of H & R Block, the income tax specialists. In the late 1980s, Richard was diagnosed with what was said to be "terminal and untreatable" lung cancer, caused by many years of smoking. His surgeon told him to go home and get his will and estate together, because there was no hope. Well, that was not the answer he wanted to hear. Richard and his wife, Annette, furiously researched the disease. Because of its reputation and willingness to help him, he checked himself into M. D. Anderson Cancer Center. After undergoing radiation therapy, chemotherapy, surgery, immune-system stimulation, and psychotherapy, Richard learned that his condition was indeed treatable. "There is no type of cancer for which there is no treatment and there is no type of cancer from which some people have not been cured," he insists.

There is a lesson in Richard Bloch's story for all of us. Asking for a second opinion should never make you feel uncomfortable in any way. Whenever cancer is involved, the situation is serious. Sometimes even a third or fourth opinion is necessary before you feel secure about both the diagnosis and the prescribed treatment. Most doctors welcome the support of their peers. If the opinions differ, the only thing that should matter to any doctor is your health. If you don't understand the diagnosis and/or treatment you've been prescribed, you will never be able to fight with the determination and gusto needed to beat this disease. Just think, after literally receiving the death sentence from one physician, Richard Bloch has had many more years of quality life and is still going strong. Doesn't that sound like a great reason to ask for a second opinion? Today, in an effort to reduce the high cost of medical treatment, many insurance companies insist on and pay for a second opinion before agreeing to underwrite any form of treatment at all.

Teamwork

The most important aspect of establishing a successful doctor/patient relationship is teamwork. I can't stress it enough. The reason cancer is such a dangerous disease is that it is difficult to control. Knowing exactly what is going on and having a say in your treatment is the only way of getting back some of the control your cancer has taken away. Regardless of how brilliant a reputation a doctor has established, if the doctor did not allow me to be a partner in my treatment, I'd find a new one. I think you should, too. On the other hand, you can't be a good partner unless you make an effort to gain as much knowledge as you need from as many sources as possible. Many doctors have gotten into the habit of making all the decisions because *we have allowed them to make all of our decisions.* If you feel your doctor is worth keeping, but he doesn't know how to make you a partner, *teach him.*

Dr. Marc Lippman describes doctor/patient relationships this way: "Imagine you are in a department store and the clerk seems anxious to help you, knowing and expecting you to be a motivated buyer. He or she seems willing to walk the aisles with you, explore the drawers and bins for obscure merchandise, or call the warehouse to see if there is anything new on order which might suit you better. This is the spirit you should expect from your doctor." Genuine concern for your recovery, genuine desire to find the most appropriate form of treatment for your particular case, and genuine likability—it's not too much to ask.

CHAPTER SIX

Knowing Your Treatment Options

Once you have been diagnosed with breast cancer, you must find out what all your options are so you can discuss them intelligently with your doctor, your family, and your friends. But before you and your doctor can discuss the options, you must both be aware of the specifics of your particular cancer, what stage it is in and how far, if at all, it has metastasized (spread). Your doctor will recommend other tests such as X rays and blood tests, and surgical removal of some or all of the underarm lymph nodes to determine just how far your breast cancer has progressed.

A chest X ray will check to see if the cancer has spread to the lungs and bone X rays will look at the ribs, back, hips, and other parts of the skeleton. The blood tests will determine the status of the liver, kidneys, and other organs. You should ask your doctor what X rays and

I very sincerely wish you would exert yourself so as to keep all your matters in order yourself without depending on others as that is the only way to be happy and to have all your business in your own hands.

MARTHA WASHINGTON

blood tests he or she is recommending, what information he or she hopes to obtain, and, after completion, what the results of these tests have shown.

One of the most important factors in determining the stage of the cancer is whether or not the underarm, or axillary, lymph nodes have been invaded by the cancer. This information is obtained by surgically removing some of the lymph nodes. If you have a mastectomy, some of the lymph nodes are routinely removed along with the breast. If you have a lumpectomy, the lymph nodes under the arm are removed by a separate incision. In either case, the physician will know if the lymph nodes are involved and, if so, how many.

The following staging system is used to describe the progress of breast cancer.

- *CARCINOMA IN SITU (CIS)* a non-invasive cancer where the tumor cells are confined to the duct or lobule, with no evidence of microscopic invasion to the surrounding tissue. Lobular CIS appears to be a marker for high risk for developing invasive cancer in either breast. Ductual CIS might be associated with the development of invasive cancer at or near the biopsy site.
- *STAGE I:* means the tumor is no longer than two centimeters (about one inch) in diameter and has not spread (metastasized) outside the breast or to the lymph nodes.
- *STAGE II:* means the tumor is from two to five centimeters (approximately one to two inches) and/or has spread (metastasized) to the lymph nodes under the arm.
- *STAGE III:* means the cancer is larger than five centimeters (more than two inches) and involves the underarm lymph nodes to a greater extent and/or has spread to other lymph nodes or other tissues near the breast.

A mammogram is crucial in detecting and defining cancers of various sizes.

Carcinoma in situ, DCIS comedo type, a very early breast cancer, side view.

Stage I breast cancer, side view.

Stage II breast cancer, spiculated mass with calcification

Stage II breast cancer.

Photos courtesy of Dr. Phil Evans

- *STAGE IV:* means the cancer has metastasized to other organs of the body, most often the lungs, bones, liver, or brain.

Standard Treatments

There are four standard forms of treatment for breast cancer: surgery, radiation therapy, chemotherapy, and hormone therapy. Beyond that, there are other experimental or neoadjuvant treatments being researched, such as bone marrow transplants. Surgery and radiation are local forms of treatment, affecting only the cells in the treated area. Chemotherapy and hormone therapy are systemic forms of treatment, affecting cancer cells and noncancerous cells throughout the body by circulating through the bloodstream and the lymphatic system. In order to treat all aspects of the disease, doctors often prescribe a combination of treatments. Usually, surgery is the primary treatment or initial treatment, and the other three are used as follow-up or adjuvant therapy. However, in some cases chemotherapy might be given prior to surgery to reduce the size of the tumor. The course of treatment your doctor suggests will depend on several different factors such as tumor type, stage, and location, your age, and your medical history.

It is standard today to be treated by a team of medical experts including a medical oncologist, a surgeon (or a surgical oncologist), a radiation oncologist, and a pathologist. (A pathologist studies tissue removed from your body to determine if cancer cells are present, and if they are, what kind of cancer cells.) You might not actually see all these people, but they will be working together to determine your treatment.

Your personal feelings about each treatment option, and how it fits in with your lifestyle and your self-image, are immensely important. Be honest with your doctor and tell him or her exactly how you feel as you discuss each possibility.

Surgery

Surgery is most often the primary treatment for breast cancer. Its purpose is to remove the cancer and ultimately stop the local growth of the disease before it has the chance to spread. If you are a Stage IV cancer patient, surgery might not be recommended, depending on the extent to which the cancer has spread. This does not mean that there isn't a treatment for you; it only means that surgery would not be in your best interest as, once again, the purpose of surgery is ultimately to prevent the disease from spreading beyond the breast to other parts of the body through the lymphatic system and the bloodstream. If your breast cancer has significantly metastasized, there is no point in putting your body through the trauma of surgery.

There are several types of surgery now commonly used in treating breast cancer. You should discuss all of them thoroughly with your A Team and decide together which procedure best fulfills your medical and psychological needs. Naturally, the first question most women have is, *Can my breast be saved?* This is a normal question, an understandable question, but should be second to the question, *Can my life be saved?*

TYPES OF SURGICAL PROCEDURES
- *RADICAL MASTECTOMY:* removal of the entire breast, the underarm lymph nodes, and the major and minor pectoral muscles and the lining over them. My Aunt Rose had a radical mastectomy, also known as the Halsted radical mastectomy (named after the doctor, William Halsted, who developed it in 1882), and if you recall, she was terribly disfigured. Although this operation was standard procedure for about seventy years, it is rarely performed in

this country anymore unless the breast cancer has spread to the major pectoral muscles.

- *MODIFIED RADICAL MASTECTOMY:* the removal of the *entire* breast, some of the underarm lymph nodes, and the lining over the chest muscles. The chest muscles are left intact, making it easier to flex and rotate the arm during and after recovery. The modified radical mastectomy is also a vast improvement over the radical mastectomy because when the major chest muscles are left in place, a woman has much more freedom of movement, her surgery is not as obvious while wearing a prosthesis, and reconstruction is more cosmetically effective.

- *MODIFIED RADICAL MASTECTOMY FOLLOWED BY IMMEDIATE RECONSTRUCTION:* A number of women are choosing to have reconstructive surgery at the time of their mastectomy. The woman should thoroughly discuss this option with both her surgeon and her plastic surgeon for complete details. More discussion of reconstruction appears in chapter 7.

- *LUMPECTOMY (Partial Mastectomy) FOLLOWED BY RADIATION:* also known as a wedge excision. This breast-conserving procedure removes the cancerous tumor plus a rim of surrounding normal tissue. Surgery is followed by radiation therapy. A separate incision is made in the axilla (underarm) area for the lymph node dissection, i.e. removal of several lymph nodes. In some early cases, the removal of lymph nodes is not necessary. For example, some in situ carcinomas (early stage cancer) are only treated with lumpectomy or lumpectomy with radiation.

If there is lymph node involvement, additional therapy will probably be required, such as chemotherapy and/or hormone therapy. The advantage of the lumpectomy is that the breast is saved, often making the disease

psychologically easier to handle. An important consideration in determining the appropriateness of this type of
surgery is the woman's breast size and the amount of tissue to be removed. For example, a small-breasted woman
might not have a good cosmetic match to the remaining
breast. Other contraindications to lumpectomy include
early-stage pregnancy; two or more tumors in more than
one quadrant of the breast; a tumor larger than five centimeters; inflammatory carcinoma (an aggressive form of
breast cancer); collagen vascular disease (an auto-
immune disease not effectively treated with radiation);
and a history of high-dose radiation to the chest or breast.
Studies have shown that the majority of women with
early-stage disease—stages I and II—treated by breast-
conservation procedures and radiation have the same survival rate as women treated with mastectomy.

- *QUADRANTECTOMY FOLLOWED BY RADIATION*: This
  procedure involves removal of a quarter of the breast containing the tumor plus some skin and the underarm
  lymph nodes. This surgery is usually accompanied by
  radiation therapy. Like the partial mastectomy, the quadrantectomy might be beneficial to large-breasted women
  in saving their breast, but for smaller-breasted women,
  this procedure will not have a pretty cosmetic result. It is
  not preferred treatment.

CONSIDERATIONS
When determining your surgical, or primary, treatment, two factors are taken into consideration above all others: first, which
form of surgery will most likely ensure your best chance of recovery, and second, which form of surgery will most likely give the
best possible cosmetic results (appearance). Although modified
radical mastectomy is the most common surgery, lumpectomy

Lumpectomy and underarm lymph node removal, the most common form of breast preservation.
(Photo courtesy of Dr. George Peters)

Modified radical mastectomy, currently the most common form of breast cancer surgery, followed by breast reconstruction with tissue expansion.
(Photos courtesy of Dr. John Bostwick)

Patient before and after, mastectomy and immediate reconstruction with implants.
(Photos courtesy of Dr. John Bostwick)

followed by radiation is being performed more often. Studies have shown that the majority of women with early stage disease—stages I and II—treated by breast conservation procedures (lumpectomy) and radiation have the same survival as women treated with mastectomy. For some, the fear of losing a breast can be more traumatic than the fear of cancer itself. This fear is what keeps many women from mammography screening and from practicing breast self-exam. For that reason alone, the advancement of the lumpectomy has been invaluable. Knowing that the discovery of breast cancer does not have to mean the automatic loss of the breast might bring more women to a psychological place where they can be aggressive about their breast health.

However, two women with the exact same size cancerous lesion will not necessarily benefit from the exact same surgery. Remember, I had a very small malignancy in my left breast, but because of its location, a lumpectomy was not my best option. The cosmetic results of a lumpectomy would have been more disfiguring than those of a modified radical mastectomy followed by breast reconstruction. A woman with very small breasts or a tumor located close to the nipple has to think carefully about what procedure will be better for her in the long run. Sometimes even if a lumpectomy is a clinical option, it is not the best cosmetic option.

As you can see, the surgical options you have are quite varied. Which surgery is right for you will become obvious after discussing your test results with your team of doctors.

Radiation

The purpose of radiation therapy is to destroy, by the use of high-energy X rays directed to a particular location, any remaining cancer cells in the breast or lymph nodes that were not removed during surgery. Whereas at one time radiation therapy was used mainly to treat patients with advanced cancer, now, with the development of the lumpectomy and other breast-conservation operations, radiation has proved quite successful as adjuvant therapy in the early stages of breast cancer. *Lumpectomy without radiation therapy is a poor choice of treatment.* There is as much as a 40-percent chance of cancer recurrence if the lumpectomy is performed without the radiation follow-up. Today, chemotherapy and hormone therapy are also considered to be adjuvant therapies after surgery, and some physicians will prescribe a combination of several different treatments when the size, location, and aggressiveness of the cancer warrant it.

If you and your surgeon have opted for lumpectomy and radiation therapy, it is very important to see the radiation oncologist (a physician who specializes in the use of high-energy X rays to treat cancer) in consultation before your surgery. Because the radiation oncologist will be providing X ray treatment after the surgery, it is necessary for him or her to be in complete agreement that you are a good candidate for this form of therapy.

After your surgery and lymph node removal are completed, you will need a week or two to heal and prepare emotionally for the next round of treatment. Your first visit to the radiation oncologist will not entail any treatment at all, but rather give you an opportunity to discuss your treatment plan openly and ask any questions you might have regarding the procedure. Together you and the doctor will discuss how the radiation will be given, where exactly the radiation will be given, and how many treatments will be required. Usually, radiation treatments are given five days a week, for five or six weeks straight.

Also during that first visit, ink lines are drawn on the body to mark the exact area that the radiation will be aimed. Do not attempt to wash or scrub the lines off because following the ink lines is the only way to be sure that the treatment is delivered in the exact same area every day. Eventually, the ink will fade. The room in which the radiation will actually be administered can be a bit intimidating at first. You will lie on a composite, nonmetallic table under a large machine—a linear accelerator—from which the radiation is dispersed. The technician will spend as much time as it takes to ensure that you are in just the right position. It is of the utmost importance that you do not move after you have been correctly positioned because the entire procedure would be useless if the radiation misses the intended tissue. The technician will then leave the room to avoid exposure to the radiation and you will be observed through a closed-circuit television. The radiation therapist will consult with the dosimetrist, the person who computes and regulates the radiation dosage. The standard dosage administered to the entire breast for early stage breast cancer is somewhere between forty-four hundred and five thousand centigray. (One centigray equals one rad.)

Radiation therapy does not hurt, but there are a few common side effects you might or might not experience in the treated area such as itching, redness, tanning, or a sunburn-like effect. The treated area might also become firm and/or rough to the feel. Many women are fatigued during radiation therapy, so it is important to get enough rest and to eat nutritiously in order to keep up your strength. Each of these side effects can be annoying, but they will pass when your treatment is completed. There are a few more serious side effects which are far less common. Because the lungs, heart, and ribs are located in such close proximity to the breasts, they unavoidably receive minimal amounts of radiation. Although it happens rarely, this exposure can cause radiation-induced pneumonia, pericardial effusion, which is fluid around the heart, or rib fractures.

As is the case with any breast cancer treatment, radiation can fail to stop the recurrence of the cancer, requiring a mastectomy at a later date. However, studies show that most women treated for breast cancer by primary radiation therapy after lumpectomy are as pleased with the outcome cosmetically as they are with the improved survival rate and prognosis.

RADIATION BOOST

In addition to the initial forty-four hundred to five thousand centigray given to the entire breast, almost all women will receive what is called a booster dose of radiation to the primary site, either externally using an electron beam or internally using an iridium implant. The external booster is being used more often these days, but the implant is still used occasionally. The purpose of the booster is to give the original tumor site additional irradiation before ending the treatment. It is, in fact, a precautionary procedure which attempts to ensure that all the cancer cells have been destroyed.

The beam boost is produced through a type of linear accelerator machine, very similar to the one used in the original treatment, aimed directly at the site of the original tumor. It will require five consecutive days of treatment. If you have your boost by beam, do not be concerned if you see additional redness or irritation; this is quite normal.

The implant procedure will require a short hospital stay, probably no more than two or three days, and is done usually under general anesthesia. Thin plastic tubes are threaded through the tissue where the original tumor was taken out. How many tubes are used depends on the size and location of the tumor that was removed. To make sure that the tubes are correctly in place, a chest X ray will be taken. Then you will be taken back to your room, where the radioactive material (iridium) is inserted into the plastic tubes.

During these two or three days, you will receive approximately two thousand rads to the site of the original tumor and surrounding tissue. The procedure is not painful, although you might experience slight discomfort at the time the tubes are being put in place and removed, much like the feeling of stitches being put in and taken out. This discomfort can be minimized with medication.

You will not be confined to your bed but will be able to move around the room freely. It is necessary to stay in a private room because the implant emits small amounts of radiation which might possibly put other people in the room at risk. Visitors must stay at last six feet away and it is not recommended that children or pregnant women enter the room at all. This is just a precaution, as the amount of radiation received by visitors is not thought to be large enough to be a health risk. After the two or three days, the plastic tubes will be removed and you will be discharged from the hospital.

CONSIDERATIONS

You will probably have a lot of questions about radiation before you can commit to this form of treatment. Just the name alone can be frightening. Here is a list of possible questions you might want to ask during your initial consultation. There are probably other questions you will want to add to the list. Ask as many questions as you need, and keep asking until you have enough information to make an informed decision.

1. What is radiation therapy?
2. After reading my pathology report, viewing the slides, and examining me, do you feel the size, location, and type of tumor I have will be responsive to radiation therapy? Will you explain why (or why not)?
3. How does the radiation work?
4. Are normal tissues damaged in the process?

5. How many treatments will I have and what is the radiation dosage I'll receive?

6. What is the course time and dosage of radiation therapy?

7. How often will I be seen by a physician during the course of treatment?

8. What kind of machine will be used? What are its advantages and disadvantages?

9. How reliable is the machine? How often is it unable to function? How old is the machine?

10. Who administers the treatment? If it is a technician, how experienced is he or she? How closely is he or she supervised?

11. How long does each treatment take?

12. Should I come alone, or should a friend or relative accompany me?

13. What side effects might occur, and how long do they last? Which side effects should be reported to the doctor or nurse?

14. Would any special diet or dietary supplement eliminate or lessen the side effects?

15. Are follow-up visits with a physician necessary upon completion of therapy? How often are checkups and tests required after completion?

16. I understand that ink markings can leave residue on clothing. Can I use tattoos, if I prefer? What does tattooing involve?

17. What are the precautions or prohibitions during and after treatment (e.g., use of skin creams and lotion, underarm shaving, etc.)?

18. Is it all right to continue normal activities such as work, sex, and sports during and after treatment?

19. How soon should treatment begin? What are the risks if I delay or miss a treatment?

20. Do you recommend other forms of treatment in conjunction with radiation therapy? Why (or why not)?
21. What is the cost of radiation therapy? Is it usually covered by medical insurance? (Check your own policy's terms.)

Chemotherapy

Chemotherapy is the treatment of cancer with cytotoxic drugs—that is, drugs that literally kill fast-growing cells, which is what cancer is all about (a short, uncomplicated definition of cancer being the rapid, uncontrolled, abnormal growth of cells). Since chemotherapy is a systemic treatment—the drugs circulate in the body through the lymphatic system and the bloodstream—unlike surgery and radiation, it can reach tiny cancer cells called "metastases." While some of these metastases might be detected by X rays, CT scans, bone scans, or physical examination, often (particularly in the early stages) they might be undetectable by currently available tests. For this reason, chemotherapy is invaluable as a weapon against cancer. Today, it is being used earlier and earlier in cancer treatment in addition to surgery and radiation in the attempt to prevent or postpone a cancer recurrence. This early use of chemotherapy is called "adjuvant" (given in addition to surgery and radiotherapy). Chemotherapy has also been successfully used to shrink large breast tumors that have not spread to other parts of the body, which allows a woman more surgical options.

Chemotherapy can be administered into a vein (IV) (either one in the arm or through a specialized type of venous access catheter—there are several types of these and you should ask your doctor), or orally through pills.

Like every other form of cancer treatment, however, chemotherapy has its own set of disadvantages. Because it cannot, as of yet, distinguish between fast-growing cancer cells and fast-growing "normal" cells in the body, there are many potential side effects associated with chemotherapy. The most obvious are loss of hair, loss of energy, nausea, vomiting, and susceptibility to infection. There are others, as well, which might or might not occur depending on your particular prescription and dosage, such as deterioration of bone marrow, mouth ulcers, rashes, changes in skin pigment, blood in the urine caused by bladder inflammation, lung damage, and weakness of the heart. And like any other form of cancer treatment, there is always the possibility that chemotherapy will not work—in this case because the cancer builds up resistance to the drugs.

Experiments and studies are being done every day to improve the effectiveness of chemotherapy while diminishing its side effects. There is also a great effort being made to simplify the form of treatment so that women on chemotherapy can continue with their regular lifestyles as much as possible.

TYPES OF CHEMOTHERAPEUTIC DRUGS

There are many different drugs used in a variety of combinations being employed to treat all kinds of cancer. The good news is that many of these drugs are effective in treating breast cancer. Let's go over each of them so that when you and your oncologist discuss them, they won't seem completely foreign.

- *ALKYLATING AGENTS*: kill tumor cells by interfering with the cells' building blocks, called DNA. Examples of alkylating agents are melphalan (Alkeran), cyclophosphamide (Cytoxan), chlorambucil (Leukeran), nitrogen mustard (Mustargen), and Thiotepa.

- *PLATINUM DERIVATIVES*: are a new family of drugs that also interfere with DNA and have activity against breast cancer. Examples are cisplatinum and carboplatinum.

- *PLANT ALKALOIDS*: also work on keeping the cells from dividing. These chemotherapeutic agents, which come from the periwinkle plant, have proven effective in treating breast cancer. Some examples of plant alkaloids are vincristine sulfate (Oncovin) and vinblastine (Velban).

- *TAXANES:* a new plant alkaloid—Taxol (paclitaxel), which originally came from tree bark and is now synthesized, is another new drug with anti-breast cancer activity.

- *ANTIMETABOLITES:* work by interfering with the cancer cell's ability to produce RNA and DNA and are especially effective in killing dividing cells. Examples of antimetabolites effective in treating breast cancer are 5-Fluorouracil (5-FU) and methotrexate.

- *ANTIBIOTICS:* have a completely different meaning when being used in the treatment of cancer than when used in the treatment of infections, because in this case the antibiotics destroy tumor cells, not bacteria. Doxorubicin (Adriamycin) and mutamycin (Mitomycin C) have proven particularly effective in treating breast cancer.

These are just a few of the most common drugs you are likely to hear about when discussing chemotherapy; you might hear others. Try not to be alarmed by the sound of their names. Remember, scientists and doctors have a language of their own. Each drug has its specific purpose and you have a right to know exactly what is going into your body and why. If you don't understand what a term means, don't be embarrassed to ask. Without having made a scientific study of the names of drugs, how are you to know what they mean? Another point to know is that chemotherapy is usually given as combinations of drugs, particularly when it is used as an "adjuvant." Several common combinations include "FAC" or "CAF" (5-FU + Adriamycin + cyclophosphamide), "AC" (Adriamycin + cyclophosphamide), "CMF" (cyclophosphamide + methotrexate + 5-FU). These combinations use several drugs to attack the cancer cell simultaneously and are usually more effective than one drug alone.

CONSIDERATIONS

I believe to get the best results from chemotherapy, a woman must receive it early in the treatment course and to maximum dosage.

"There is good data today on the amounts of drugs that are effective. A few years ago there was controversy over the use of chemotherapy (particularly combination chemotherapy) to treat breast cancer, both in the adjuvant setting and for metastatic disease. Many excellent clinical trials have shown both the benefit as well as the limitations and toxicities of chemotherapy. Breast cancer is a complex and multifaceted disease and thus the results from these studies that apply to your case must be sorted out by your physician as they learn the specifics of your individual case. From this they can give you information based on scientific knowledge about the likely benefits and toxicities for chemotherapy and hormonal therapy for you. Factors such as your tumor's stage, receptor status, DNA content, lymph node involvement, as well as your age, menopause status, other medical conditions, family, social, and job factors, will all enter into the decision. You must participate in the decision with your doctors to decide whether chemotherapy or hormonal therapy are right for you," said Dr. John Minna, University of Texas Southwestern Medical Center.

It is also very important to know that the team of doctors, nurses, and pharmacists have become very skilled at giving the chemotherapy to minimize its side effects, while maintaining its anti-cancer activity. For example, considerable care goes into the preparation of individual IV doses of drugs by the pharmacist. The use of catheters makes blood access and IV infusion less painful. The doses are carefully calculated based on body height and weight and adjusted if unnecessary side effects occur. The blood counts are carefully monitored, and hormones to stimulate blood cell production can be used. Both can reduce the chance of infection from low blood counts; and most important, anti-nausea agents (anti-emetics) are now very effective at greatly decreasing the vomiting and nausea that used to always occur with chemotherapy.

I wish there were a way to eliminate it, but right now losing your hair is a frequent side effect to chemotherapy. All forms of chemotherapy are cytotoxic. If you have made the commitment to go through the treatment, why not fight the disease with the most powerful weapons available in full dosage?

The side effects of chemotherapy are almost always temporary, but occasionally they aren't. It is a risk every cancer patient must face. I personally think the risk is worth taking. Only when we see confirmed proof that milder dosages of chemotherapy are as effective as the strongest dosages in preventing a breast cancer recurrence, will I support them.

However, you have to make your own choices. Sometimes the quality of life, even in shorter time increments, is more important than the quantity of life. This largely depends on the stage of a particular cancer, the age of the patient, and the patient's lifestyle. What was right for me might not be right for you. We all have to respect the individual choices made by each cancer patient. I just want to make sure that every woman with breast cancer understands the seriousness of the disease and is aware of all the options from which she can choose. Breast cancer is a formidable opponent. To win the war, you *have* to *fight.*

Here is a list of common questions most often asked when chemotherapy is prescribed. Use it as a guideline and add to it whatever you need in order to have a better understanding of your treatment.

1. What, specifically, is chemotherapy, and why is it indicated in my case?

2. What is the significance of lymph node involvement in relation to chemotherapy?

3. How many of my nodes were involved?

4. What were the results of my hormone receptor assays and my flow cytometry test? What other tests did you run? How did the results of these tests influence your treatment suggestions?

5. Which chemotherapy drugs are you recommending for me? Why have you chosen those particular drugs rather than another combination?

6. How many months will I need this treatment?

7. How frequent are the treatments?

8. How are the drugs administered?

9. Will I have to go to the hospital for treatment?

10. How long does each treatment take?

11. Should I come alone for the treatments, or should a friend or relative accompany me?

12. Tell me all the possible side effects I might experience. Are they permanent? Does everyone get them?

13. Is there anything I can do to lessen or relieve the side effects?

14. How much do these treatments cost? Will they be covered by my health insurance?

Chemotherapy has proven its effectiveness in putting some cancer patients in complete remission. Other times it doesn't work at all; still other times it can add a few good years to a woman's life. To me, knowing all the risks, enduring this often unpleasant form of treatment was worth every minute of suffering I experienced, though at times during the treatment I might not have admitted it. You must think about all the benefits, weigh them against the negatives, and decide for yourself what is best for you.

Hormone Therapy

Like chemotherapy, hormone therapy is a systemic treatment. Unlike chemotherapy, it is not cytotoxic—it does not kill cancer cells directly. Hormones are substances naturally produced by the endocrine glands. Their purpose is to stimulate other organs. Hormones are largely responsible for reproductive functions (such as ovulation and milk production) and for aspects of appearance that distinguish the sexes. When cancer begins in tissues that are affected by hormones, such as the breasts, it is possible the tumor will be affected by hormones as well. In premenopausal women, drugs that suppress female hormones (estrogen and progesterone) might also suppress the growth of cancer. In postmenopausal women, other types of hormones might have the same effect.

Originally, hormone therapy as a treatment for breast cancer was limited to the surgical removal of hormone-producing glands, as in an oophorectomy (the removal of the ovaries). Today, however, while surgery to remove the ovaries might be desirable in treating cases where the production of hormones by the body is believed to be speeding up tumor growth, synthetic drugs such as tamoxifen, megestrol acetate, or aminoglutethamide plus hydrocortisone have been proven to control recurrent breast cancer and produce long remissions from the disease as well. Once again, the names of the drugs are more intimidating than the drugs themselves. The truth is that in many cases where hormone therapy is an option, the side effects are much less troublesome than with chemotherapy. In rare cases, however, hormone therapy might cause serious side effects such as depression, blood clots, or rarely, elevated levels of calcium in the blood. Very rarely, hormone therapy produces the opposite effect from that intended and the tumor growth is speeded up. Tamoxifen is a very widely used synthetic drug which acts to block the binding of estrogen to its receptor in breast cancer cells, and in so doing dramatically blocks the growth and potentially kills breast cancer. It is often used as an adjuvant therapy and can be combined with chemotherapy. Because of its benefits as an adjuvant therapy, there is a large clinical trial going on called the Breast Cancer Prevention Trial to determine if tamoxifen could prevent the development of breast cancer in women who are determined to be at high risk. Patients taking tamoxifen have a small risk of developing a type of uterine (endometrial) cancer. Although tamoxifen somewhat increases your risk, it is important to remember that *all* breast cancer patients—not just tamoxifen patients—are at greater risk for uterine cancer. When your physician recommends tamoxifen it is because he or she believes that the benefits of reduced risk of relapse and prolonged survival outweigh the risk of uterine cancer. We anxiously await the outcome of the Breast Cancer Prevention Trial.

One problem with hormone therapy is that it can take up to several months to determine whether or not it is having a significant effect on the tumor. Therefore, if your cancer is posing a threat to a vital organ, chemotherapy would have to be used instead, since it works much faster.

It is crucial that a hormone receptor assay be done at the time of biopsy to determine whether or not hormone therapy is an option for you, and that you be made aware of the results. The presence of estrogen and progesterone receptors in breast cancer is thought to be associated with high survival rates and long-term remissions. However, if your hormone receptor assay proves to be negative, as was mine, you can still achieve optimal results through chemotherapy and/or radiation in conjunction with your initial breast surgery. Clearly, the best advantage of having a positive hormone receptor assay is that it gives you another option in treatment.

CONSIDERATIONS

Here are some questions you might want to know the answers to before considering hormone therapy. As always, use them along with your own questions.

1. What is hormone therapy?
2. What were the results of my hormone receptor assays?
3. How and why do they warrant this treatment?
4. Which hormone drugs are you recommending for me, and why?
5. In what form will the treatment be given, and how often will treatment be given? How long will treatment take?
6. Should I have hormone therapy in conjunction with any other forms of treatment?
7. What if hormone therapy does not work for me? What other choices do I have?
8. What are the side effects I might encounter and what, if anything, can I do to prevent them from occurring?
9. What is the cost of hormone therapy, and will it be covered by my insurance?

New Approaches to Treatment

Now that we have discussed the standard cancer treatments, let's talk a little bit about treatments we are *not* sure of at this time: biological therapies, clinical trials, bone marrow transplant, and the so-called "alternative therapies."

Biological Therapy: The New Frontier

I refer to biological therapy as the new frontier in breast cancer research because it is exciting and offers hope for the future. Through the study of what they call biological response modifiers, scientists are now beginning to understand cancer at its most basic cellular level. This means they are getting closer to discovering what causes a normal cell to change into a cancer cell. To me this sounds like a great breakthrough. I can't help but wonder, however, what will happen thirty years from now if, in a moment of rare nostalgia, my son Eric should pick up this book with his own son or daughter and glance through the pages. Do you suppose they'll laugh at what I once thought was a great breakthrough? Probably.

Immunotherapy means just what the name indicates—an effort to stimulate the body's immune system in order to recognize and attack cancer cells. Today it is still highly experimental, though progress is being made in all forms of systemic adjuvant therapy. New substances are being tested every day. The important and positive aspect of immunotherapy is that it has been sometimes noted to benefit the advanced cancer patient as well as patients who have detected their cancers early.

Perhaps the greatest hope for the treatment of breast cancer in the future will come from therapies that are based on an improved understanding of the way in which breast cancer begins and progresses. Dr. Marc Lippman offers us the simple yet useful analogy of asking a cave man to try to stop a car's engine. If he takes out a club, there is no question that sooner or later he could get the car to stop, but by then the car would be reduced to a complete wreck. While this might be an overstated analogy for chemotherapy and radiation treatment, it is also clear that these therapies can damage normal as well as abnormal parts of the body. A more rational understanding of how a car works leads to half a dozen strategies which could conceivably stop the car without damaging it, such as turning off the ignition, siphoning out the gas, pulling off the distributor cap, etc. In the same sense, as we start to understand the specific components that set a cancer cell apart from normal cells (its ability to grow continuously in an unregulated fashion, its ability to invade normal structures and tissues, and finally, its ability to break away from the parent tumor mass and spread throughout the body), we will be able to design therapies that are directed against these factors.

Great progress has been made in the last few years in understanding the changes in DNA (mutations) that occur in breast cancer cells in very specific genes that change the normal cells into cancer cells. These genes are called dominant and recessive ("tumor suppressor") oncogenes. An example of a dominant oncogene involved in breast cancer is the Her-2/neu gene. Some new treatments specifically directed against Her-2/neu are already being tried. Examples of recessive oncogenes are the p53 and BRCA-1 genes. A clinical trial to vaccinate breast cancer patients against a mutant p53 gene is already underway.

Another benefit from studying recessive oncogenes is that they can be used to trace breast cancer in families. Pioneering studies by Dr. Mary Claire King at the University of California at Berkeley showed that a predisposition to breast cancer can sometimes be inherited. Dr. King pinpointed a gene (BRCA-1, which stands for **Br**east **Ca**ncer gene #1) that has recently been isolated ("cloned"). With the specific DNA sequence in hand, it will now be possible to sequence DNA from members of some breast cancer families and see which women inherited the mutant, cancer-causing gene.

In order for the BRCA-1 gene to cause cancer, an alteration or mutation must be present. Since it is such a large gene, finding the mutation is difficult and time-consuming. Mutations might be different in different families, adding to the difficulty of isolating the alteration or mutation and developing tests to determine risk.

Scientists are hopeful that genetic testing will be available soon at the research level to a small number of families participating in familial breast cancer research and for whom a linkage to BRCA-1 gene has been detected. Dr. Francis S. Collins at the National Institutes of Health directs the Human Genome Project, an international effort to locate and map human genes. The work being done on this project, and other worldwide projects, is at the forefront of finding a cure for breast cancer.

"While there are many social, legal, and ethical questions to answer in addition to knowing how to use the information to help individual women, this is a very exciting area to help with breast cancer early detection and prevention," said Dr. John Minna, University of Texas Southwestern Medical Center.

The Komen Foundation is currently funding genetic research in the laboratory as well as in a clinical research setting. Dr. Mary Claire King of the University of California at Berkeley is a Komen research grant recipient. Her genetic research discoveries have been of major significance in unlocking critical genetic information in the progression of breast cancer. UT Southwestern Medical Center in Dallas is using Komen grant funds for its Familial Cancer Registry which identifies and monitors people who have an increased risk of cancer due to familial background.

We don't yet know how much breast cancer occurs due to family inheritance. In addition to BRCA-1, the p53 gene can be inherited in a mutant form to give an increased risk of breast cancer (and other cancers). A BRCA-2 gene was just recently reported.

There are undoubtedly several more such genes that scientists will find over the next several years. Because this is an evolving field, if you have a family history where several members have cancer (even other than breast cancer), children with cancer, or several female blood relatives with breast or ovarian cancer, you should try to get into a family cancer registry so, as this new technology develops, it can be used to help you and your family. You can call a comprehensive cancer center in your area to determine if there are local clinical trials in which you might be eligible to participate. Or call the Komen Foundation National Tollfree Breast Care Helpline at 1-800 I'M AWARE (1-800-462-9273) for more information.

Clinical Trials and Research Studies

Clinical trials and research studies involving patients with breast cancer are important sources of information on new treatments. Much of what is used successfully in the treatment of breast cancer today comes from the clinical trials conducted in years past. These successes are in large part due to the courageous women who participated in past clinical trials. It is essential that these valuable clinical trials continue to be supported so that medical science can move closer to finding a cure. Clinical trials are important and should continue to be supported.

I was lucky. I was placed in a clinical trial that has proven to be very successful. If I had to make a choice about whether or not to participate in a clinical trial again, I would do it in a heartbeat. Some women feel that being a part of a study group makes them a "guinea pig" for scientists; I disagree. Today, medical science has become so advanced that you will always be given some form of studied treatment which will be matched against another form of proven treatment to see if there is a slight or marked edge for one over the other.

You can find out what clinical trials are being done, and where, by contacting PDQ (Physicians Data Query), a computerized information service that provides doctors and patients with the most up-to-date cancer information possible. PDQ can tell you who has the state-of-the-art facilities and where the newest tests are being conducted (see Resource section). When you call,

you will need to know your diagnosis, including type and stage
of cancer, where the primary cancer is located, cell type, and
address and phone number of the physician who is providing
your treatment. The information PDQ gives you, however, is
written in medical terminology that most of us will not be able
to understand. It is better to tell your doctor that you have
accessed PDQ and have the report sent directly to him or her.
You can then go over the information together. (See Resource
Guide, page 231.)

The NSABP

For many years a wonderfully dedicated man, and my good
friend, Dr. Bernard Fisher, headed the National Surgical
Adjuvant Breast and Bowel Project. The NSABP is one of the
nation's oldest and largest ongoing cancer clinical trials. It is
sponsored by the National Cancer Institute and involves some
five thousand physicians at more than four hundred sites in the
United States and Canada.

Beginning in 1958, the NSABP brought together a group of
surgical oncologists to investigate adjuvant therapy for breast
and bowel cancer. Adjuvant therapy is treatment such as radiation or chemotherapy used as a supplement to the primary form
of treatment, which is surgery. This group pioneered the now
well-established breast-conserving procedure of "lumpectomy
followed by radiation" as an alternative to "mastectomy."

Through years of study, the NSABP has concluded that there
is equivalent survival for the procedure of "lumpectomy followed by radiation" as compared to mastectomy. Lumpectomy
followed by radiation allows breast cancer patients to keep their
breast. According to the American College of Radiology and the
American Cancer Society, at least one-third, and perhaps as
many as one-half, of all breast cancer patients could have a

choice in how their cancer is treated. Breast cancer patients should talk with their doctor about treatment options in order to make informed decisions.

In 1992, the NSABP began a large Breast Cancer Prevention Trial to study the anti-estrogen drug tamoxifen as a preventive agent for breast cancer in women who are healthy but at high risk of breast cancer. Data of women *with* breast cancer who have taken tamoxifen for two to five years indicates a 40 to 50 percent lower incidence of a second breast cancer. This is encouraging information for the participants in the Breast Cancer Prevention Trial. The drug tamoxifen might also lower the risk of heart disease and osteoporosis.

Because of the pioneering work of Dr. Fisher and his colleagues, these and other studies done by other cooperative groups offer more treatment options for breast cancer patients and greatly improve the quality of life for breast cancer survivors.

Bone Marrow Transplantation

Another promising approach in breast cancer treatment is bone marrow or stem cell transplantation. In this procedure, your bone marrow cells are collected from your hips, or, with the newest techniques, in some cases taken from your own blood stream, and stored away. Actually, this is not a "transplant." Rather, it is the storage of your blood-forming cells so that you can be given very large amounts (so-called "dose intensive") of chemotherapy and then be given back your own marrow or your own stem cells to rescue your blood-forming system from the massive therapy. Currently, this very intense and costly therapy is being tested in clinical trials particularly on women who at diagnosis have a large number (greater than ten) of lymph nodes involved with breast cancer. Bone marrow transplantation is the subject of much controversy and we will have to await scientific data to know how frequently it will be of benefit. If you are considering such therapy, you should only make the decision after extensive consultation and be treated at a center specializing in such therapy and participating in clinical trials.

Alternative Therapies

Rose Kushner once said, "Remember, today's quackery may be tomorrow's breakthrough!" Of course, she was referring to the fact that scientists might be open-minded but need to prove theories with hard research and testing. As a member of the National Cancer Advisory Board, I had the distinct privilege of meeting some of the most respected scientists in the country. I have sat in on numerous panel discussions and have witnessed firsthand the genuine thrill that is felt when a breakthrough is made. I have also been around when what was thought to be a promising discovery fails in some way—everyone mourns. There is no hidden cure for cancer. When the cure *is* found, the whole world will know about it. The National Cancer Institute is always willing to listen to new ideas about breakthrough possibilities. However, all hypotheses must be tested and proven in the same strict format as is used in any other practical study. The health and safety of all people depend on it.

Alternative therapies are treatments for cancer that have not been sanctioned by the medical community's clinical trials—for example, vitamin therapy, coffee enemas, a macrobiotic diet, an all-fruit diet, homeopathic medicine, and laughter therapy. I investigated the subject with a number of doctors and some of my associates on the National Cancer Advisory Board. Just about every physician I spoke to admitted that most of their patients "do something" in addition to conventional medicine. And why not? Why shouldn't you do anything and everything you can to make yourself feel better? The problem begins when people attempt to *replace* conventional treatment with these alternative therapies.

However, although proper diet, the right vitamins, some natural herbs, and exercise are certainly helpful in keeping the body clean, fit, and healthy, so far, none of them has been proven to successfully stop or even slow down cancer. The isolated cases you might hear or read about are not, I believe, something to pin your hopes on. One to two percent of all cancer patients go into what is called spontaneous remission, cancer remission without the aid of medicine. When this happens—and it is rare—the situation is the exception, not the rule. Please don't be fooled into thinking a crazy diet or a mysterious herb is going to cure your cancer.

A woman I know who has been a good friend for a long time developed a small breast cancer and was successfully treated and reconstructed. A beautiful, energetic woman, she seemed to handle her illness with a great attitude and recovered quite quickly. She was a role model to other cancer patients. Speaking to women's groups about her experience, she helped many women. A year and a half later, my friend was diagnosed with a kind of lymph node cancer called lymphoma. Her doctor advised her to undergo chemotherapy, feeling her chances for a possible long-term remission were excellent. What happened between her recovery from breast cancer and her development of lymphoma, I'm not sure, but now she wanted no part of chemotherapy or any conventional medicine. She opted for a strict macrobiotic diet as her sole treatment. Afraid that she would be criticized by her friends and doctors, this woman checked into a rather well-known "cancer clinic" over the border. Well, her disease did not regress; instead, it had spread throughout her body. My friend died before this book was published.

Perhaps none of us really knew how the treatment for breast cancer affected her. Maybe her side effects were worse than she ever let on. My friend had no children and had been through a painful divorce. She had no one for whom to fight. I feel that because she was an educated cancer patient, she simply opted for the quality of life rather than the quantity and knew in her heart what the outcome would be. I really don't believe she actually thought this diet would take the place of medical science. Still, it was her choice to make and we all must respect that whether we agree with it or not. I'm just sad because I loved this friend.

On the other hand, I am in full agreement with trying anything and everything to make the unpleasant experience more tolerable as long as your doctors are aware of what you are doing and it does not interfere with the primary and adjuvant cancer treatments. During my courses of chemotherapy, I found imaging particularly helpful. I tried to look at "the big picture" first, thinking that these few months of sickness would be minuscule compared to the rest of the healthy life I intended to live. At the times when it got really bad and I felt so sick, I thought back to childbirth. *That* was much worse. Before each treatment session I would plan a fun outing for a few days afterward. It didn't have to be anything fancy—a movie with Eric or a quiet dinner out with Norman would do just fine. When I started to feel bad, I would visualize myself already there, and I would feel better right away.

I also surrounded myself with a lot of "white light," meaning a lot of positive energy. I tried to be with only people I knew cared deeply for me and for whom I cared deeply. I read poetry and listened to soft music. When I felt up to it, I took long walks in the sunshine and rode horses. I tried to meditate and made it a point to be thankful for my blessings. Above all, I never discounted the power of laughter or the power of prayer. Spiritual and religious awakening is a subject that is current and exciting. If you are interested, there are wonderful books describing how to enter a state of personal fulfillment or spiritual peace. I highly recommend them. You can find them in the metaphysical studies or new age section of a bookstore.

In Summary

The important thing to know about any and all forms of cancer treatment is that *you have choices*—no matter how far your cancer has progressed.

Surgery, radiation therapy, chemotherapy, and hormone therapy are constantly being tested and retested for ways of improving the process, and promising and exciting new ways of treating breast cancer are continually being studied. Research your disease. Talk to your A Team. Talk to patients. Call the Susan G. Komen Breast Cancer Foundation National Tollfree Breast Care Helpline at 1-800 I'M AWARE (1-800-462-9273).

CHAPTER SEVEN

Breast Reconstruction

There are some women who choose never to have reconstruction following mastectomy. Going through surgery and/or radiation and chemotherapy might be all the trauma they would like their body to endure. Other women feel that they cannot get along without it. Knowing that reconstruction will bring back her feminine silhouette might be the determining factor in a woman's decision to go through with the mastectomy.

> *It's always something.*
> GILDA RADNER

Clearly, the decision to have reconstructive breast surgery is very personal and depends on several important factors including age, general physical health, and self-image. Having had breast reconstruction two years after my mastectomy, I feel the best thing about reconstruction is its ability to promote a sense of wellness. Although I adjusted well psychologically to losing a breast, got used to wearing a prosthesis, and was successful in getting back to a normal life, my missing breast was a constant conscious and subconscious reminder that I had had cancer. It wasn't until after my reconstruction that I could truly begin to put the disease behind me. On one level the fact that I have had breast cancer will never be completely forgotten. In the back of my mind there is always a thought of recurrence—that's the negative. However, because my own life was threatened, I will forever appreciate the fact that I am alive and healthy—that's the positive. But now even though it is my chosen career to talk about breast cancer, there are some days that go by in which I honestly forget to include myself as someone who has had the disease. That never happened before my reconstruction. Of course, there were other benefits to this surgery as well. I can wear just about anything I like and I no longer feel lopsided when my bra comes off. For me, breast reconstruction was the right choice. For you, it might not be.

If you are considering this surgery for yourself, you need to know what it entails. There are two major types of reconstructive surgery: immediate—at the time of mastectomy—and delayed—performed months or years after the mastectomy. *Talk to your surgeon about it before your mastectomy, if possible,* because he might tell you that you are a candidate for immediate reconstruction, or if not, the position of the mastectomy incision might affect the later reconstruction procedure.

If you have already had a mastectomy and are just now considering the option of reconstruction, don't worry. Almost every breast cancer patient is a candidate for reconstruction. Scarred, radiation-damaged, grafted, thin, or tight skin, and even the absence of chest muscles no longer prevent reconstruction.

Talking to other women who have gone through the surgery will help you get a new perspective if you are unsure about the procedure. Try to find women of approximately your own age to talk with, as their questions and thoughts might be similar to yours. If you can't find anyone, call the American Cancer Society's "Reach to Recovery" program (see Resource Guide, page 231).

Choosing a Reconstructive Surgeon

The most important factor in choosing a reconstructive surgeon is finding someone who is experienced, and technically and medically competent. It is also important to find a physician who is thoughtful and understanding of the psychological impact breast surgery of any kind has on a woman. Your oncologist and/or surgeon might be helpful in giving you some names of reconstructive surgeons to interview. Or consult the American Society of Plastic and Reconstructive Surgeons (see Resource Guide, page 232).

When talking with the surgeon, discuss your feelings about the procedure openly and candidly. This will help you decide if you are comfortable talking to him or her and able to establish the necessary rapport. Ask to see photographs of the surgeon's work and get the names and phone numbers of some of his or her other patients.

Here is a list of questions that might help you get started in your interviewing process. You will probably have many more to add to this list. As always, you should continue to ask questions until the procedure is clear in your mind.

1. What type of reconstructive surgery do you recommend for me, and why?
2. What types of implants are available and are they safe?
3. What are the risks and benefits associated with this type of surgery?
4. How much experience have you had with this type of surgery?
5. May I see photographs of other patients who have had the various types of reconstruction?
6. May I speak with other patients about the procedure?
7. What can I expect my reconstructed breast to look and feel

like after surgery? How, if at all, will this change in six
months or a year?

8. How long will I be in the hospital?
9. How long is the recovery period following surgery?
10. What should I do or avoid doing to ensure a safe and fast
    recovery?
11. How soon can I have this operation?
12. What else should I consider before committing to recon-
    structive surgery?
13. What about my other breast?
14. How do you get a mammogram after reconstruction?
15. How much will it cost? Will this operation be covered by
    my insurance?

When Should Reconstruction Be Performed?

The trend in recent years has been toward immediate reconstruction. Several influences have made this possible. First, skin-
sparing mastectomy procedures have become more common
and this additional available tissue facilitates more predictable
artistic results. Second, adjuvant therapy (treatment in addition
to surgery) has shifted away from radiation and toward
chemotherapy. While radiation significantly compromises the
immediate reconstruction, chemotherapy does not. Finally, as
reconstruction becomes accepted as a routine part of the treatment, it is more efficient for the patient to start it at the time of
the mastectomy.

With the controversy over the safety of silicone, many
women are now afraid to have implants. The preference for
reconstructive methods using natural tissue, usually from the
abdomen or back, has grown rapidly. A further refinement in the

use of natural tissue has been the expanded use of microvascular transfer techniques. This involves attaching blood vessels from the transferred tissue to blood vessels in the chest wall.

To determine what is appropriate for you, I suggest you discuss all the variables with your oncologist, your breast surgeon, and the reconstructive surgeon you have chosen. Together you should be able to come up with a plan that fits both your personal needs and your medical needs.

Types of Reconstructive Surgery

There are three common procedures used in breast reconstruction. As in all types of breast cancer treatment, each woman's case is individual and the procedure that is the best for you should be discussed thoroughly before a final decision is made.

Skin Expansion Plus Implant

When minimal skin needs to be removed with the mastectomy, a temporary *skin expander* might be placed as the wound is closed. Over a several-month period of office visits, the expander is inflated to slowly stretch the mastectomy skin to the size of the remaining breast. Once stretching is complete, the temporary skin expander can be replaced with a permanent breast implant. The nipple reconstruction is most often performed at the second step when the permanent implant is inserted. Silicone gel implants are no longer available, but saline-filled implants can be used.

Transverse Rectus Abdominus Myocutaneous Flap (TRAM)

To create a chest muscle and breast mound, the surgeon transfers one or both of the patient's two abdominal rectus muscles,

Patient following mastectomy.

Patient after reconstruction using Skin Expansion Plus Implant. Reduction surgery on opposite breast. Nipple reconstruction.

Patient before mastectomy and reconstruction surgery.

Patient one year later after Latissimus Dorsi reconstruction and nipple reconstruction.

Patient with Latissimus Dorsi scar.

Photos courtesy of Dr. Fritz Barton

Side view of patient following mastectomy.

Front view of patient following mastectomy.

Ninety-degree side view of patient nineteen months after reconstruction using TRAM flap (Transverse Rectus Abdominus Myocutaneous Flap). Nipple reconstruction and reduction of opposite breast. Abdominal scar and resulting "tummy tuck."

Front view of patient nineteen months after reconstruction using TRAM flap (Transverse Rectus Abdominus Myocutaneous Flap). Nipple reconstruction and reduction of opposite breast. Abdominal scar and resulting "tummy tuck."

technically called Transverse Rectus Abdominus Myocutaneous, from the stomach to the chest. This procedure is commonly called a "TRAM." This flap of muscle, skin and fat is shaped into the contour of the opposite breast. If there is enough abdominal tissue available, no implant is needed. This procedure also tightens the abdominal muscles, giving rise to the term "tummy tuck" procedure. The patient will have a scar across the lower abdomen in addition to the mastectomy scar on her chest. Because there are, in effect, two surgeries being performed, recovery might be prolonged.

Latissimus Dorsi Flap

This procedure is used when the TRAM procedure is not an option. To create the reconstructed breast, the surgeon transfers skin and muscle from the patient's back (this muscle is called the latissimus dorsi) to the site of the mastectomy. The reconstructed breast might require an expander or implant if there is not enough tissue to reach the proper volume. In addition to the mastectomy scar on the chest, the patient will have a scar on the back. (See the photographs on page 151.)

In both types of Flap reconstruction, the flap may be moved to the breast site while still attached to the patient's blood supply; or as a "free flap" where this tissue is separated from the patient's blood supply, moved, and reattached using microsurgery.

Nipple Reconstruction

New techniques have greatly improved nipple reconstruction. The most common current method is to surgically create a prominence to resemble the nipple by combining little pieces of tissue (skin and fat) from the dome of the reconstructed breast mound. This is called the "modified skate flap" and is done in a second surgery. The timing of this surgery will depend upon the healing process of your original surgery. Pigmentation for the new prominence or nipple and the surrounding areola is done in a subsequent procedure and is usually achieved by medical tattooing. This is done as an office procedure.

In Summary

For some women, breast reconstruction has a profoundly positive psychological impact. For other women, it is an unnecessary extravagance. And then there is the consideration that it is a major operation requiring general anesthesia. The decision is one that requires a lot of research and discussion. Whether you choose one of these procedures or not, it is important that you know they exist. A major part of being a strong, aggressive cancer patient is understanding all of your options.

CHAPTER EIGHT

Appearance and Recovery

There is probably no other time in a woman's life when she feels less like making herself look attractive than while she is being treated for cancer, yet I know of no other time when the effort is more rewarding. That effort includes paying attention to your makeup and wardrobe, and exercising to keep your body attractive, too.

> *Do wear makeup— it's so vain not to.*
>
> COCO CHANEL

I have seen and spoken to many breast cancer patients over the years. Some of the women I have spoken to have had early-stage breast cancer, others have been more advanced. I have noticed a certain pattern in the women who have had success in their treatment. They seem to be a little more vain, a bit more concerned about self-image, and a little more willing to do whatever it takes to preserve that image than the women who weren't as successful.

But beauty is more than the way you look. It is also the way you view life. A woman who always sees the bright side is often considered more beautiful than her negative counterpart, regardless of what she actually looks like. This is not to say that one should "view the world through rose-colored glasses." The ability to see things exactly the way they are and yet find the best in even the worst situation is indeed a gift—*one that can and should be cultivated.*

Still, almost everyone will agree that when you look good, you feel better. I know several women who have been in the depths of cancer despair and no one would ever have known it to look at them. Mary Tullie Critcher, a board member of the Komen Foundation and a cancer patient, is one of those women. I distinctly remember her coming to a meeting immediately following a chemotherapy treatment. Most women in her condition would not have shown up for the meeting at all. But Mary Tullie was there, looking more beautiful and more pulled together than ever before. She was wearing a soft, silky scarf on her head over which she wore a wonderful hat that matched her dress. The look was quite chic. Mary Tullie is a typical American wife and mother. What inspired her to make such a noble effort?

"My family was very upset and frightened by my illness," Mary Tullie explained. "When they saw me looking as if I felt good, they believed I was getting better. The doctors and nurses at the Medical Center also seemed to get a lift when I showed up for a checkup or a treatment looking well. Other patients, too, took note of my scarves and hats, wanting to know where they came from or how I did it. Pretty soon, if even for just a short while, I forgot how sick I was."

Another very special woman is the late GiGi Hill. GiGi was given less than a 5 percent chance of living five years after being diagnosed with metastatic breast cancer in 1980. Knowing exactly what the odds were, GiGi made up her mind that she was going to live those five years with style and grace. She never missed a charity event, never missed a party, was always there for her family and friends, and always looked divine. She took the time to see that her makeup was applied beautifully and that her wigs were always in place. In October 1985, GiGi was given the Betty Ford Award at the Komen Awards Luncheon. She marched up on that stage in front of some fifteen hundred people, shook Mrs. Ford's hand, and flashed her most gorgeous smile. The audience went wild. No one could have guessed from her appearance that she was only days away from death.

Taking the time to make yourself look as good as possible will help you get through your illness. When you look sick, people are bound to inquire about it—that's human nature. If everyone you meet asks you what's wrong, *it will be difficult to get past your illness and get on with your life.* By dressing and living every day as normally as you can, you will be giving your subconscious mind the message that you are "healthy." To paraphrase a friend: What the mind believes, the body tries to accomplish. So, think, talk, and act in positive and optimistic ways.

Taking the time to make yourself look as good as possible will also do wonders for your morale. I guarantee it. There are all kinds of uncomplicated tricks you can use to make the process easier and more successful. Several of them I learned through my own experimentation. Some I picked up from other cancer patients, and still others I found out about through the "Look Good...Feel Better" program sponsored by the Cosmetics, Toilet and Fragrance Association in partnership with The American Cancer Society. (See Resource Guide, page 231). They worked for me; I hope they'll work for you.

Hair

The most traumatic aesthetic side effect of cancer treatment is, of course, the loss of hair (alopecia). Your hair surrounds your most prominent means of communication, your face—no wonder it is so important. For most women, the possibility of going around without hair is unthinkable. Scars from surgery can be concealed without anyone knowing about them. Covering a bald head is more difficult. I found the wigs that look the most natural to be the most time-consuming and difficult to put on. Wearing the obviously fake hair was hassle-free, but I had to realize that strangers would know I was sick. It didn't matter—I wanted to get on with my life. The good news is, hair loss due to chemotherapy is almost always temporary. Also, not all women lose their hair. In the meantime, you can hide your loss by wearing wigs, scarves, and hats. Use the time to experiment with different styles and/or colors. Making the most of this emotional trauma will do wonders for your morale.

Wigs

In choosing a wig for yourself, try to go to a person or wig salon specializing in the needs of chemotherapy patients. This is a very emotional and vulnerable time for any woman, and the last thing you need is an insensitive salesclerk pushing a product that is simply not you. Make sure that wherever you go has a place you can be helped in private. Sometimes an owner will open the salon at "off" hours to ensure your privacy, or if you are really lucky, you may find someone who will come to your home.

Shop for your wig *before* beginning chemotherapy. The salesperson can see your hair color, your particular style, and you can try on different styles to see which one you like best. You might want to take a friend along when you go, or your hairdresser if that is possible.

Wig salons today sell excellent synthetic wigs that look and feel like real hair, but are easier to manage and are a fraction of the cost of natural wigs. Natural wigs are expensive and difficult to manage. They need setting more often, usually at a salon; the color will fade and require salon treating. Depending upon the length you choose, an excellent synthetic wig will start at approximately one hundred fifty dollars. The synthetic wig is permanently "set" and you can wash it yourself and style it with a comb and brush. But remember, since your wig is synthetic, avoid extreme heat such as steam, curling irons, or blow dryers. Your wig salon will give you a pamphlet with complete care and setting instructions.

Obviously, what you are striving for is to look as normal as possible. I cut my hair short before I started with the chemotherapy so the change would not seem as drastic to me. Many women find it easier to make the adjustment from short hair to no hair, rather than from long hair to no hair. Some salons suggest that cutting long hair prior to hair loss reduces the weight pulling at the hair, making hair loss less noticeable.

It is difficult to get a true fit for a wig until you have lost all your hair, although you may want to have the process organized and ready before that time. If you choose a wig before you've lost your hair, ask if you can leave a deposit and pay for the wig later, when you are sure the fit will be correct. If you opt to wait until you can ensure the perfect fit, bring with you a couple of photographs with your hair looking just the way you like it. That way the specialist can do his or her best to make you look as close as possible to the way you are used to seeing yourself.

The concern of every woman who purchases a wig, regardless of the reason, is that it will stay in place. There are several products on the market to ease your anxiety. Wig caps are made of nylon stocking material and help hold the wig in place. They sell for approximately five dollars. Wig liners are made of cotton and serve the same purpose, but can also be used as sleeping caps. They sell for approximately fifteen dollars. The cotton sleeping cap is a wonderful idea, for without the protection of hair, your head will get quite cold.

In addition to the wig caps, you may purchase a wig band that has a strip of Velcro sewn onto it. The wig is placed over the band and adheres to the Velcro. You can also purchase a two-sided adhesive product that helps hold your wig in place. This product is similar to those used by men who wear hairpieces. However, if you choose to use these strips, you should take extra care when removing the adhesive piece. You may risk skin irritation or infection.

When selecting a wig color, most salons suggest you opt for one as close to your own hair color as possible. This will make the transition much less noticeable. After your initial wig purchase, you may want to consider buying a second wig, if that is financially possible for you. That way, while you are washing, drying, and styling your original wig, you will have an extra to wear.

Although at this point in your life you are purchasing a wig out of necessity, remember that most of the wigs sold are to women who have hair. Wigs today are quite versatile and very fashionable. Try to make this experience as fun as possible and experiment with different looks. And remember, it is only temporary.

A note about insurance: Although every insurance company has its own rules and regulations about what is and isn't covered, most consider the loss of hair as they would the loss of a limb requiring a prosthesis. Have your physician write out a prescription for a "wig prosthesis" and make sure your wig salon uses the word *prosthesis* on the sales receipt so that it is not confused with a wig purchased for cosmetic reasons. Check the *Yellow Pages* of your phone directory under Wigs, taking care to choose one that specializes in serving the medical patient. If you are unable to afford a wig, contact Y-Me, an organization which maintains a wig bank for women with financial need, or the American Cancer Society's "Reach to Recovery," who may be able to help. See the reference section at the end of this book for telephone numbers.

Scarves and Hats

Scarves are a terrific alternative to wigs. They are fast, simple, and stylish. You can purchase scarves in a variety of different textures and colors to complement any outfit. They should be cotton rather than silk or polyester, as these materials have a tendency to slip around on the head. The best size to use is either a twenty-six- or a twenty-eight-inch square. There are dozens of different ways to tie scarves into interesting headwraps, ranging from very conservative to very avant-garde. Most any department store or accessory store will have books on how to tie scarves. Take advantage of them. The important thing is to develop a style you are comfortable with. Many times, the look is so fabulous, women keep right on wearing scarves long after their hair returns.

Hats can be an equally charming touch to complete an outfit. Most hats don't cover the entire head, however, so it is important to wear them over a scarf. Berets and caps will give you a sporty, fun look; fedoras a more classic, conservative look; and wide-brimmed hats will protect your skin, which will be extrasensitive at this time, from the sun and wind.

Turbans are a very fashionable alternative to the scarf or hat. A consultant at a shop specializing in wig needs for medical patients gave me a great piece of advice. She said to invest in a "bang" hairpiece to wear under a turban or scarf. That way, if you have put on your makeup, added some jewelry and the bangs, you will look like you are wearing the turban or scarf by choice and not by necessity.

As I have said throughout this book, do your best to *look* good, even though you might not feel like expending the effort. It will make you *feel* good.

Skin

Any authority on beauty will tell you repeatedly that even the strongest, thickest skin should be treated delicately. Skin that is being subjected to radiation and/or chemotherapy can be especially tender and sensitive. Be gentle. When washing your face, use a liquid or cream cleanser; they are less harsh than soap. Even if your skin is oily, it is still extra-vulnerable right now. Look for an oil-free cleanser and then follow up with an astringent or whatever your regular routine involves.

Some women find that while going through radiation and/or chemotherapy, their skin is dry, red, irritated, or a combination of any of these, even when normally it is on the oilier side. Moisturizers, skin lotions, and body oils will take away the dry, irritated, chapped feeling caused by your treatments. Occasionally, the skin will react to the fragrance in some of these products. If this should happen to you, don't despair—you will not have to give them up. Almost every major cosmetic and toiletry company makes a line of products that is fragrance-free. If you are going through radiation, there might be certain restrictions to what you might apply to the area being radiated, so consult your physician.

Because your skin is sensitive, take your baths and showers in water that is warm rather than hot, especially if you are receiving radiation or have undergone breast reconstruction. After reconstruction the breast area is numb and has no feeling. Be especially careful to avoid hot water.

If you are experiencing hair loss from chemotherapy, be sure not to neglect your scalp just because there might be little or no hair on your head. If you suffered with the problems of dryness, itching, and dandruff before your hair loss, you will suffer with them during and after your hair loss as well. It is thought that a daily massaging will stimulate blood flow in the area and might produce a stronger, healthier, and shinier head of hair after chemotherapy.

Sun

By now we have all heard about the damage too much sun can do to the skin. Despite the warnings of skin cancer and premature aging, however, many women still find it necessary to spend countless hours in the sun during the summer and never miss a day in the tanning booth during the winter.

It is especially important while you are undergoing cancer treatment to be careful of sun exposure. Too much sun while taking certain chemotherapy drugs can cause permanent changes in the skin pigment.

Still, having a "healthy glow" will be the first thing you, your family, and your friends will look for as proof that you are well on your way to recovery. Using a sunscreen of SPF (sun protection factor) 15 or higher will keep you safe from the sun's harmful rays (if applied faithfully every two hours and after swimming) and still allow a slow tan. If you want to look healthy but refuse to submit your skin to potential sun damage, don't forget the wonders of makeup. You might also want to try the self-tanning creams that are available. They work wonderfully well. However, check the label to see if they contain a sunscreen. If they do not, you will need to apply sunscreen if you are going to be in the sun for an extended period of time. Follow the guidelines of the American Cancer Society by avoiding the sun during its most harmful hours and wearing protective clothing.

You should also be aware that radiated skin will always be extra-sensitive to the sun. So please take the proper precautions. If you are in any doubt about your personal exposure to the sun or the use of any cosmetic products, always consult your physician.

Makeup

Carefully applied makeup can be very helpful at this time. For some women experimenting with cosmetics is fun, and trying to make yourself look healthy at this time presents an interesting challenge. Even if you have always detested wearing cosmetics, you might want to give them a try. Maybe you've thought the look was unnatural or perhaps you've never wanted to take the time and trouble. You are not alone. Many women prefer a more natural look and feel to their skin. But now, while you are experiencing some of the side effects of breast cancer treatment, the "natural look" might not be the most flattering. Temporary changes in skin color can make you appear yellow, gray, washed-out, pale, or in some cases, flushed and ruddy. You might be experiencing puffiness and either complete or partial loss of eyebrows and eyelashes. A little bit of knowledge on just the basics of makeup artistry can give you the lift you need. Most of the aesthetic side effects of chemotherapy and radiation can be corrected with cosmetics.

Changes in skin color can be corrected with such products as foundation and under-eye concealer. If your skin has turned gray or yellowish, wear a foundation with a rose or pink hue. On the other hand, if you are experiencing a ruddy, red tone in your complexion, wear a foundation with a peachy hue. This will counterbalance the temporary color change. Dark circles under the eyes can be virtually eliminated with under-eye concealer. There are many different formulas of this product with many different consistencies.

If your eyebrows have fallen out, either completely or partially, don't use eyebrow pencil to fill them in. Eyebrow pencil has a tendency to look harsh and phony. Using a powder eyebrow color allows you to recreate the look of eyebrows in a much softer, gentler manner.

Every woman wants to have long, lustrous eyelashes; chemotherapy can take that dream away for a little while. Wearing false eyelashes can help recreate the look. I found, as have many cancer patients and noncancer patients alike, that the individual lashes are far more natural-looking than the strip lashes. Once you get the hang of it, these individual lashes are a cinch to apply. You can wear them by themselves or to supplement any existing lashes. And if you use a good glue, they can stay in place for weeks, looking fabulous.

These are actually only a few of the many tricks cosmetics can do for you at this special time in your life. If you are not comfortable playing with the products, treat yourself to a makeover. At a local department store, there is usually no charge for a cosmetic makeover, but in most cases, there is little or no privacy. If you go to a private salon, the cost will be anywhere from forty to two hundred dollars, but you will be helped by a licensed cosmetician who might be more familiar with your particular needs. Another option would be to call the headquarters of one of the direct sales cosmetics companies such as BeautiControl or Mary Kay Cosmetics. They will put you in touch with a consultant in your area who will come to your home for a private consultation. Even if you are an expert at makeup application, it is sometimes fun to see what someone else might do with your face.

Remember that seeing you look good is equally important to your friends and family as it is to you—sometimes more so. Do make an effort to look your best, even if it's just a little lip gloss and blusher—for their sake.

Dressing

The two most common treatments for women with breast cancer that affect clothing are the mastectomy and the insertion of a subclavian catheter. Also, of course, there is a short time after a lumpectomy and/or biopsy that you might feel a little sore or uncomfortable, but that should pass within a week or two.

The good news is that today a woman can dress very casually and comfortably, and still be considered chic and fashionable. At one time, sweat suits were worn only in the gym, but now they can be worn almost anywhere. Even with dressier clothes, more attention is paid to comfort now than ever before.

When dressing immediately after surgery or to cover a venous access device, try to wear blouses that are loose-fitting. The catheter sits right below the clavicle (collarbone) and halfway between the neck and shoulder. Big, soft collars will cover the area without causing any discomfort. Scarves strategically thrown over the shoulder will also help camouflage the catheter. Shoulder pads lift the fabric away from the body, keeping the area free from abrasion.

Breast Prostheses

If you have had a mastectomy, you will need to wear a breast prosthesis, which is an artificial device replacing your breast. Besides the obvious advantage of making the body look "normal," the prosthesis will keep your body weight balanced.

Without the prosthesis in place, your upper body will be lopsided, which could cause a great deal of discomfort in your back, shoulders, and neck. Today, breast prostheses have been revamped for the active woman. They can be worn doing almost anything, even swimming. And, they can be worn with just about any type of outfit except, of course, one that shows cleavage.

Get the "okay" from your physician before being fitted for your prosthesis. The physician will want to make sure the scar has healed and all swelling has gone down. You might want to use one of the soft, unweighted dacron breast forms until you can be fitted for a permanent prosthesis.

There are different types of prostheses from which to choose, and they slip into a pocket sewn into your bra or swimsuit. You can even get some that adhere to the chest wall and can be kept in place for several days. You will want to go to a prosthesis shop to try on the latest types. The kind you will find most comfortable will be based on your bra size, cup size, and the actual shape and weight of your other breast. Here are a few recommendations you might want to consider:

- Check with your insurance carrier or Medicare/Medicaid to determine what insurance coverage you have.
- Try on several, from different manufacturers. They all fit a little differently, so you will want to get the one with the best fit and feel for you.
- Wear a form-fitting top when trying on the prosthesis.
- Wear the prosthesis for about half an hour while in the prosthesis shop.
- It is also a good idea to check the return policy of the prosthesis shop before purchasing.

At night, many women wear a sleep form to bed because the back, neck, and shoulders are susceptible to the same strain lying down as they are standing up and moving around. The sleep forms are not as heavy as the silicone forms worn during the day. They are usually made of polyester, cotton, or foam.

Your emotional recovery walks hand in hand with your personal self-image. Your comfort plays a large role in how you feel and the speediness of your ability to get back into the mainstream. For this reason, it is imperative that in being fitted for your prosthesis you seek the advice of a qualified expert. Look in the *Yellow Pages* under "artificial breasts" or "prosthetic appliances," or contact the local chapter of the American Cancer Society's "Reach to Recovery" program at 1-800-ACS-2345. The Y-Me organization maintains a prosthesis bank for women with financial need. Call 1-800-221-2141.

Exercise

There is no question that a mastectomy is major surgery. Besides making you feel lopsided there is a great deal of discomfort and stiffness involved. Fortunately, having a mastectomy rarely causes any permanent limitations in movement, and often, steady exercise can speed up your recovery. However, women who have lost their chest muscles through a radical mastectomy (very uncommon today) might not regain 100 percent of their original strength in the affected arm and shoulder. Still, a regular exercise routine can alleviate some of the tightness in the chest.

Exercise, as was proven in my case, is also very helpful in relieving the symptoms of lymphedema, which is the swelling of the arm following the removal of the lymph nodes in the armpit (axilla).

No exercise program should be contemplated or begun without the expressed consent and guidance of your surgeon. Your surgeon or physician will recommend specific exercises depending upon your type surgery. You might also contact the "Reach for Recovery" program of the American Cancer Society for exercise information (see Resource Guide page 231). As soon as your physician gives you the go-ahead, a low-key exercise regime should be your next physical goal.

The key is to exercise only to the point where it begins to feel uncomfortable—don't push yourself. Remember, regular exercise will speed your physical recovery, which will enhance your appearance and benefit your emotional recovery.

Emotional Recovery

To all of the tips above on prostheses, wigs, makeup, clothing, and exercise, one more must be added. There's a risk factor in your emotional recovery: depression. Depression is anger turned inward. Depression, if it strikes, can cause you to say, "Why bother taking care of myself?" The good news is that there are people who can help you overcome this problem, too. I know the diagnosis, treatment, and recovery from breast cancer is a stressful period for you and your loved ones. To help you cope through this time, it might be important to seek professional support. Support groups, led by knowledgeable professionals, bring people together to share common experiences. In addition to open discussions where group members share feelings and talk about their progress, most groups also have planned educational sessions. Group facilitators are professionals who have expertise which enables them to provide vital resources and answer your questions. There are even support groups for children and spouses.

Call the American Cancer Society "Reach to Recovery" program, Y-Me, or The Susan G. Komen National Tollfree Breast

Care Helpline at 1-800 I'M AWARE. See the Resource section for telephone numbers. There are understanding, caring people at these organizations who can assist you in finding the help you need. Take advantage of them. You deserve it.

℮

CHAPTER NINE

Sexuality

Self-image, as it pertains to sexuality, can be a monumental issue for any woman. It is ingrained in our psyches at an early age through movies, television, books, and magazines that in order to be attractive and desirable to men, we have to have a certain *look*. Flat stomachs, shapely hips, lean legs, and full breasts are the components of a "sexy"-looking woman, so they say. This kind of pressure, we all know, is unhealthy and unfair. Men, of course, do not have a specific physical "standard of excellence" to live up to in order to be considered attractive and desirable.

A woman who has been diagnosed with breast cancer faces three major losses with which she must come to terms. The first is loss of life. The stage of her disease, her spirit and willingness to fight, and her body's ability to *work with* the prescribed treatment are all factors that will determine her prognosis. The second is the loss of her breast.

Some people are still unaware that reality contains unparalleled beauties. The fantastic and unexpected, the ever-changing and renewing is nowhere so exemplified as in real life itself.

BERENICE ABBOTT

Some women fear the loss of a breast will make them less than whole, that their altered body will prevent them from ever having a normal life again or keep them from being a complete woman. The third loss is the loss of her hair. Because 99 percent of the time hair loss is only temporary, a woman's fear of it is often dismissed without a lot of psychological evaluation. But I can tell you, through personal experience and through talking with literally thousands of cancer patients, that this fear is a real one, for a woman's hair has a significant effect on her ability to feel desirable.

Some women are so preoccupied with the thought of losing their sexuality that they will opt to forgo what could be life-saving surgery altogether. My sister Suzy is a prime example. On the day my breast cancer was diagnosed, my ultimate concern was to save my life, to get rid of the cancer as thoroughly and as quickly as possible. This was based on my fear of going through the same slow, painful death as Suzy did and the fact that I was an educated cancer patient. My priorities were pre-established. Every time I had gone in for a biopsy prior to then, I had thought long and hard about what I would do if the tumor was malignant. Still, on that evening before my surgery at M. D. Anderson, sitting in the bed looking at Norman, I quietly wondered how he would relate to his relatively new wife's coming home without a breast. My wonderful friend Sharon McCutchin called me on the telephone and, sensing my concern, said in her long Texas drawl, "Honey, don't worry about it. *That's* not what they really care about, anyway." All I could do was pray she was right.

In the two years that passed between my mastectomy and my reconstruction, I learned a great deal about the true meaning of sexuality. Once again, what works for one woman might not work for another, but I want to share this with you, with the hope of reaching anyone who can possibly benefit from my experience.

I learned that my ability to be desirable to Norman had little to do with my breasts (or lack thereof). I learned that a kind smile, a gentle touch, and a sweet conversation did more for our romance than sexy lingerie. From the day we met we had always been able to communicate. If we were going to get through this without losing the sparkle, we had to continue to talk openly and honestly about the situation. The truth is that after my surgery and the treatment that followed, quite often I wasn't in the mood for romance. It was up to me to make sure that this was not mis-interpreted as a lack of love. Norman, being the kind of man he is, understood my feelings. I made it a point to let him know how much I loved him and needed him and to show him that I was trying to get well. Whenever I could help it, and sometimes I couldn't, I tried desperately not to feel sorry for myself and to maintain a cheery disposition. Norman often expressed his pride in my fight to beat the disease. This encouragement "egged me on" and gave me the incentive to keep trying even on those days when I wanted to give up. His lack of pressure and expecta-tions of me on a sexual level made me try harder to please him.

The fact of the matter is that a mastectomy rarely affects the partner's pleasure or ability to be fulfilled sexually. It is the woman's loss of a sensitive, sexual area that might affect *her* sense of pleasure. There is no reason why, after a few initial adjustments, a couple cannot rekindle a romance that is equally as sensual and full of love as it was before her surgery. Sometimes, when two people acknowledge their own mortality, as a run-in with cancer often forces them to do, their newfound appreciation for life will bring them closer than ever before.

It is vitally important for all women before, during, and after breast cancer to take the time to re-evaluate what it means to be a "total woman." Is it the size and shape of our breasts and how we look in a bathing suit? Or is it our ability to nurture and pro-tect those we love? I have for a long time felt that women have a sixth sense, if you will, which encompasses a capability to give open and unconditional love in a deeper, more passionate manner than men will ever have. It is, I think, ingrained in women, a gift we were given naturally—something we have no control over. It is this compassion from which true sexuality is born. Of course, we all want to be thought of as attractive and desirable. But on what is this desirability based? Certainly not on our ability to fill a bra. If we do what we need to do in order to be and feel healthy—eat right and exercise—we will have the energy it takes to tackle life with spirit and grace. To me, *that's* what makes a woman sensual. Looking good is usually an added benefit that comes along with doing what it takes to feel good.

Sometimes, however, eating right and exercising aren't enough to maintain a healthy body. Breast cancer chooses its victims for no apparent rhyme or reason. The healthiest woman in the world can get breast cancer. When this happens she has new choices to make. And sometimes, one of those choices will be to have a mastectomy. If she can get herself in a mind-set to believe that her energy and spirit for living are what make her sexy, she will be much better equipped to handle the emotional and psychological stress involved in losing a breast.

The sexual problems some couples face after a lumpectomy or mastectomy are often the result of preconceived notions on the part of either partner. For example, the man is often afraid to touch the woman after surgery for fear that she might not be up to it or that he might hurt her accidentally in the process. The woman, who has probably already thought herself no longer desirable, might take his lack of overtures as the justification of her feelings. She then will be reluctant to initiate a sexual encounter out of fear of further rejection. This is a very common situation and one that can escalate way out of proportion without open and honest communication. As uncomfortable as it might be at first, it is in a couple's best interest to resume sexual activity, even on the mildest scale, as soon as physically possible. If you have tried and just can't seem to muster up the desire for sex after your surgery, or you cannot get a feeling of desire from your partner, you both might want to consider seeing a counselor to open the lines of communication.

But what about the single woman who goes through the mastectomy without a husband or partner? What happens when her surgery is complete and she feels like "getting out there" again in the dating circle? When you go through the diagnosis and treatment with a partner, regardless of the difficulties that might ensue, at least you don't have to carry the burden of a very private and personal secret a woman without a partner holds inside her waiting for the appropriate time to divulge. When *is* the appropriate time to tell a man you are dating that you've had a mastectomy? Obviously, for every couple the situation will be different. Some women like to get it out in the open at the very beginning of a relationship. Others prefer to wait and see if the relationship will progress enough to become intimate at all.

The late Sherri Firnberg, an exuberant young woman actively involved in the Komen Foundation, was at age twenty-eight bravely and optimistically beginning treatment for her second recurrence. Sherri was not married, and every time she met a new man, she went through the dilemma of when to tell him. She said, "My first choice is really to keep it a secret. It's not that I have a problem talking about the experience—I don't. But I like to let people see that I'm okay before I start to talk abut the cancer. Some people react funny when they hear the word. All of a sudden, they look at you as if you are going to fall apart right in front of them. Unfortunately, though, my secret isn't often a secret for very long. Inevitably, my date and I will run into someone I know and they'll ask how I'm doing. At that point I feel sort of obligated to tell. I did meet a man I thought was special. He turned out not to be, but when we first met, we hit it off right away and I immediately felt close to him. I ran over to his house and told him everything. I was relieved when he said it didn't bother him at all. This man was a little older than most of the men I have dated. Maybe it isn't fair to make such a generalization, but so far I have found that older men take the news much better than younger men."

It is important to handle this in a manner that makes you feel comfortable. While constantly talking about it might not be the best way to put the past behind you, your breast cancer and subsequent mastectomy are certainly nothing to be ashamed of. When the situation calls for it, speaking from your heart about your experience can help bring you close to friends in general and perhaps add an element of intimacy and closeness to conversations with potential lovers. With the threat of AIDS on everyone's mind these days, we are seeing a more cautious attitude toward sexual activity. People are taking the time, once again, to get to know each other before adding the sexual dimension to their relationships. I can't help but feel this is a good thing for all couples, but for women who are trying to decide who should know about their medical past, it is especially helpful.

Whether you are happily married, unhappily married, divorced, separated, widowed, or single, one thing is for sure: If you would like to begin or continue a successful sexual relationship, you must first be comfortable with your own self-image. Nobody can give that to you—it must come from within. Remember that dealing with a mastectomy isn't easy for anyone. Your friends, lovers, and children will take their cue from you. If you honestly believe that you are every bit the woman you were before your surgery, so will all who know you and come to know you. And perhaps, if you are lucky, you will find, just as I did, that developing the inner strength to take on cancer as an opponent gives you a sense of femininity you never knew existed. Once you learn that *real* sensuality comes from within the heart and soul, you will also learn that it can never be taken away.

CHAPTER TEN

Talking About Your Breast Cancer

A s I have mentioned earlier, talking about breast cancer can be difficult. Many people have not been brought up to discuss intimate topics with others comfortably. I know in my heart that in the beginning my own husband was not completely at ease with the subject.

> *Talk happiness.*
> *The world is sad*
> *enough without*
> *your woe.*
>
> ELLA WHEELER WILCOX

The intimacy of this disease, coupled with the fear of cancer in general, often creates a communication block within the family, among friends, and at the workplace. The stage of your cancer, combined with your prescribed treatment and how your disease responds to that treatment, will determine the kinds of challenges you are forced to meet along the way.

When and how much to tell your friends, family, and business associates are factors to be considered carefully. As a rule, I feel that honesty is, as always, the best policy. However, you will know, better than anyone else, in whom you can confide.

Having breast cancer is nothing to be embarrassed about. Being surrounded by a close support group will make the ordeal easier and less stressful. You must be prepared, though, for those who react in an unexpected manner. There are people who are still so afraid of the word *cancer* that they can't bring themselves to talk about it. This can be especially difficult. Friends, family, and business associates with whom you have always been able to communicate easily might now seem to withdraw just at the time when you need them the most. People who don't understand cancer and how its treatment works are often so afraid of *saying the wrong thing*, they might say nothing at all. You might find this very hurtful. Be patient. Those who love and care about you will also feel like victims of your disease. Their terror and anger over what has happened can manifest itself in "funny" ways.

Most people will take their lead from you. If you learn to talk honestly, openly, and optimistically about your breast cancer, they will, too. Fair or not, don't be surprised to discover that just when you need to be comforted and nurtured more than at any other time in your life, *you* are the one doing much of the comforting and nurturing. That, my friends, goes with the territory of being a woman.

You can talk about telling them you know they care and you *do* want to talk about it, or you can say, "I know you care and that you have questions, but I don't want to discuss it today." For many families, the trauma of dealing with a life-threatening disease brings them closer than ever before. My friend Chris Plunkett, a wife and mother of four older sons and a young daughter, Sarah, had breast cancer which turned into metastatic disease. She was a woman of amazing strength. Chris explained to her family exactly what was happening and they, as a group, were involved in all her treatment decisions. Young Sarah proved to be her mother's greatest inspiration. This girl wanted more than anything to have her mother there for her as she went through her teenage years and on into adulthood. Sarah educated herself about breast cancer and was quite knowledgeable about all aspects of the disease. Sadly, Sarah did not get her wish. Chris Plunkett died in 1992. Sarah still volunteers her time to the Komen Foundation, speaking to groups of all ages about what the family can do to support a mother with breast cancer. When Sarah Plunkett addresses an audience, there isn't a dry eye in the house. Another friend, Gretchen Poston, handled her situation very differently. When Gretchen was diagnosed with breast cancer, she told no one. She went through surgery and chemotherapy all by herself. On the days when the treatment was difficult to endure, she said she wasn't feeling well and stayed at home. She cut her hair short before her chemotherapy began and wore a well-made wig when her hair fell out. Afterward, when Gretchen felt up to it, she did talk about the experience. Her friends were puzzled that she hadn't taken them into her confidence. Gretchen explained that it wasn't a matter of not trusting her friends, it was just that she felt she could get through the ordeal more successfully without the pity of others. Because Gretchen was a high-profile Washington, D.C. figure, she did finally go public with her story in 1989. Gretchen lost her battle with breast cancer in January 1992. To honor her memory as the founder of the Washington, D.C. Race for the Cure®, each year the race committee gives the Gretchen Poston award to the race volunteer who goes above and beyond. In 1994, Norman's daughter, and my stepdaughter, Brenda Brinker Bottum, won that award for her work on the Baltimore, Maryland Race for the Cure®. We are both so proud of her and the work she is doing.

If you have ever attended a Race for the Cure®, you have noticed the sea of neon-pink visors scattered throughout the crowd. Every time I look at that sight I am reminded of my dear, dear friend, the late Ellen Barnett, who was willing to talk about her breast cancer and who first vocalized the need to "celebrate" survivorship. She conceived of the pink visor as a way to recognize survivors and honor them at Race for the Cure® events. At first the numbers of women willing to come forward and wear the visors was small, but as the idea took hold, more and more women survivors began to don the visors and proudly proclaim their survivorship in years, months, some even days. It is inspiring now to see hundreds of pink visors worn by smiling women who are bonded together in a sisterhood of survivorship that only those who have endured breast cancer can know. I thank Ellen Barnett for speaking out and for the gift she gave to us in this program.

As in all matters concerning breast cancer, speaking about it is a personal decision. I know that I could not have fought the disease as strongly as I did without the love and support of my friends. But there are certain times and situations in a woman's life when she might be on her own. This does not mean she can't survive the disease; there is always someone to talk to. Another reason my friend Gretchen chose to stay silent was a real concern that some of her clients might feel that she could not carry out her professional responsibilities in her business. Unfortunately, this kind of discrimination does exist. Furthermore, for some women in situations like Gretchen's, pulling the strength and courage to fight from deep inside ultimately gives them a confidence and feeling of self-worth they have never known before.

The women I know who have not only been successful in fighting breast cancer but have been an inspiration to other cancer patients, have known when to discuss their problems and when to keep silent. There is a time and place for both. Remember, there is a difference between developing the ability to talk openly and honestly about the disease and unloading your anger, fear, and confusion onto anyone who happens to cross your path. Advocacy and anger have their place in any breast cancer patient's life. I found it always helps to try to strike a balance between fighting the disease publicly, and saving enough strength for the very personal fight. Today, breast cancer is much more widely discussed, thanks to the Komen Foundation and organizations like it.

CHAPTER ELEVEN

Factors That Might Affect the Risk of Breast Cancer

I would like nothing more than to tell you exactly how to prevent breast cancer from entering your life and the lives of those you love. Obviously, I can't do that or I would have used the same preventive measures on myself. What I can tell you is what factors put women at *high risk* of contracting the disease.

Pray for the dead and fight like hell for the living.

MOTHER MARY JONES

These risk factors are to be duly noted and respected, but please, be aware of this:

- Approximately 85-90 percent of all breast cancers occur in women without a family history of breast cancer.
- Two-thirds of breast cancer occurs in women older than fifty, and much of this is not dected early   primarily because they are often not aware of their risk and therefore not as compliant with screening recommendations.
- Approximately one hundred eighty-two thousand women are diagnosed every year with breast cancer, and forty-six thousand die.
- Breast cancer will account for 32 percent of all cancers in women.

All women are at risk of breast cancer, however, some women might be at higher risk.

Known Risk Factors

- The most significant risk factors for breast cancer are *being a woman and getting older.*
- A woman who has been treated for breast cancer in one breast has an increased risk of developing cancer in the opposite breast.
- Women with close female relatives (mother, sister, or daughter) who have had breast cancer might be at higher risk than women without the family history. The risk increases if more than one close family member has had breast cancer, those breast cancers were in both breasts, or when breast cancer has occurred before the age of fifty.
- A small number of women undergoing biopsy will be diagnosed with "atypical hyperplasia." This is a condition in which there are more than the usual number of cells in a breast biopsy specimen. The cells appear somewhat abnormal, but do not meet the criteria necessary to diagnose breast cancer. These women will be at increased risk for developing breast cancer.
- Although late menopause and early onset menstruation were once thought to significantly increase breast cancer risk, the risk might be more relative to population rather than to individuals. However, this is still being researched.
- Although the incidence of breast cancer is higher in white women than in black women, the five-year survival rate is lower in black women than white women. African-Americans with breast cancer face more than twice the

risk of dying compared with white Americans, primarily because they are diagnosed at a more advanced stage. This is explained in part by lower use of early detection methods and lack of health insurance. Curiously, breast cancer incidence is higher in young black women than in young white women. The reasons for these age-related differences are not known.

- We also see families where breast and ovarian cancers cluster together, and we now know that a specific gene (BRCA1) is responsible for many of these clusters.

Having one or more of what are considered to be known risk factors does not mean you will get breast cancer. Nor does being free of risk factors mean you will not get breast cancer. These risk factors should neither frighten you nor give you undue confidence. Any woman can develop breast cancer.

Birth Control Pills

There has been a great deal of press directed to the correlation between birth control pills and breast cancer. The most reliable scientific information to date finds no consistent link between taking birth control pills and developing breast cancer. Some experts feel that each patient should be carefully examined before a determination is made as to whether she should take birth control pills. If I were taking them, I would be especially diligent about adhering to a regular routine of breast self-examination, mammography, and clinical breast examinations. However, I would, and do, recommend the same diligent program to all women, regardless of whether they take birth control pills or not.

Diet

A variety of studies looking at breast cancer incidence in the United States and other countries have pointed to an association between low-fat, high-fiber diets and lower breast cancer rates. There are published data showing that women who have had breast cancer and who eat a low-fat diet have a lower chance of recurrence of breast cancer. There is growing evidence that one's nutrition plays very heavily in the development of certain diseases. I look in the future toward more and more studies validating the preventive aspects of a healthy diet. Certainly, we are going toward a diet with less fat overall, but especially less animal and saturated fat, toward more fruits, vegetables, and grains. I truly feel nutrition is extremely important.

Following a low-fat, low-cholesterol, and high-fiber diet will decrease your susceptibility to many other medical problems as well, such as heart disease, diabetes, gastrointestinitis, fatigue, and obesity. According to the American Cancer Society, people 40 percent or more overweight increase their risk of breast and other cancers, so maintaining a healthy, desirable weight is very important. Ignoring the fact that a healthy diet can save your life is inviting trouble. The key role of diet in cancer prevention is brought into focus more clearly when you consider this: Studies have shown that a Japanese woman living in Japan (the Japanese being known for a diet which is practically fat-free) has approximately one-eighth the risk of developing breast cancer as a Caucasian American woman. But when that Japanese woman moves to the United States, within one generation her female descendants have equally the same risk of developing breast cancer as their Caucasian counterparts.

A diet rich in natural vitamins A, B carotene, and C might offer some degree of protection against breast cancer. Most

Food Guide Pyramid

KEY

● Fat (naturally occuring and added

▲ Sugars (added)

These symbols show that fat and added sugars come mostly from fats, oils, and sweets, but can be a part of or added to foods from the other food groups as well.

Fats, Oils, & Sweets
Use Sparingly

Milk, Yogurt, & Cheese
Group
2-3 Servings

Meat, Poultry, Fish, Dry
Beans, Eggs, & Nuts
Group
2-3 Servings

Vegetable Group
3-5 Servings

Fruit Group
2-4 Servings

Bread, Cereal, Rice, & Pasta Group
6-11 Servings

Courtesy of USDA, Human Nutrition Information Service

medical experts will agree that the operative word here is *natural*. For some people, taking large doses of vitamin supplements can be very dangerous because of the body's inability to excrete these supplements in a safe, timely manner. The best way to get the vitamins your body needs is to get them naturally from foods such as broccoli, carrots, spinach, brussels sprouts, cabbage, cauliflower, tomatoes, sweet potatoes, green peppers, squash, apricots, oranges, strawberries, cantaloupe, lemons, and limes.

Fruits, vegetables, and bran are beneficial because of their high fiber content. The role of fiber in reducing the risk of heart attacks has been widely publicized. Here is some information from the U.S. Department of Agriculture. In its Food Guide Pyramid, the USDA emphasizes foods from the five major food groups. Each of these food groups provides some, but not all, of the nutrients you need for a healthy diet. Good health depends upon heredity, environment, lifestyle, and the health care you receive, but following these food guidelines can go a long way. Daily recommendations include:

- six to eleven servings from bread, cereal, rice, or pasta — all foods from grains. You need the most servings of these foods each day.
- three to five vegetable servings
- two to four fruit servings

These foods come from plants and provide the vitamins, minerals, and fiber needed in your diet.

- two to three servings of milk, yogurt, and cheese
- two to three servings of meat, poultry, fish, dry beans, eggs, and nuts

These foods come mostly from animals and provide protein, calcium, iron, and zinc.

- Fats, oils, and sweets should be used sparingly, as they provide calories and little else.

General recommendations are to eat a variety of foods, choose foods low in fat, saturated fat, and cholesterol, and use sugar, salt, and sodium in moderation.

I believe that additives are going to be looked at more closely in the future, as are pesticides and other environmental substances in which we come in contact with daily. I believe the comprehensive cancer center of the future will, in addition to all the traditional treatments and techniques, employ mind/body techniques that will begin to find the growing connection between mind and body in the prevention, treatment, and cure for breast cancer. I'm convinced the mind is a powerful instrument in determining one's health.

I certainly don't have to tell you what components make up a healthy diet—you know. We all have to make our own choices. I am particularly careful about what I eat, for many reasons, the most important being the threat of a cancer recurrence. Still, I have learned to enjoy the life I have, and that includes an occasional glass of wine, hamburger, and dessert.

Smoking

Although there is no known link at this time between breast cancer and smoking, I cannot in all good conscience neglect to mention the detriments of this habit. It is the number-one cause of lung cancer deaths in the country, and lung cancer has surpassed breast cancer as the leading cause of cancer deaths in women. There are no advantages to smoking cigarettes. None.

Alcohol

There is no certain evidence linking alcohol consumption to an increased risk of breast cancer. Some studies show an association without proving causation, while other studies range from no increase in risk to those that show a 20- to 40-percent increase in risk among moderate to heavy drinkers. No studies show large increases in risk associated with moderate alcohol consumption, states Dr. Victor Vogel, M.D. Anderson Cancer Center, Houston.

Some studies show definite beneficial effects of moderate alcohol consumption on overall health. A glass of wine or other spirit per day is said to aid in digestion and contribute to the production of the "good" cholesterol, or HDL. However, it is known that overconsumption leads to liver disease. As is most often the case, moderation is always the best. Please use your own good judgment, and consult your physician if you have any questions.

Antioxidants

No doubt you have read a lot lately about antioxidants. They are mostly vitamins (such as vitamins C and E) that appear to lower the risk of developing many types of cancer. Lower risks of cancer are associated with diets that are rich with these substances. There is not yet conclusive evidence that vitamin supplements taken in addition to the diet can lower the risk of cancer, although some studies do indicate protection with some vitamin supplements.

Few studies show reduction in the risk of breast cancer among women with higher intakes of vitamin C and E. On the other hand, vitamin A and related substances do show the ability to prevent breast cancer in laboratory animals. A large study using a vitamin A derivative in Italian women with breast cancer is being conducted to prevent second breast cancers from occurring. Results should be available in a few years.

I like to think I am giving myself every edge I can, so for me personally, I take a daily multivitamin plus antioxidants. But by all means, if you have any questions, please consult your physician. He or she is your authority, the person in whom you have put your trust.

Stress and Exercise

Although there is no conclusive link to stress and breast cancer, I can't begin to tell you about the number of friends who have developed breast cancer who firmly believe stress was a contributing factor. That stress can take many forms: financial hardship, work pressures, divorce, children, to mention some of the "biggies."

The key is to try and reduce the stress in your life. It might sound selfish, but you have to *be good to yourself.* It is important to recognize when you have over-committed yourself or pushed yourself too much. Learn to pace yourself, take a break when stress builds up, and by all means, learn to say "No." You need to stay in control of your life in order to control stress. I can't tell you how important this is. There are a number of good "relaxation" tapes on the market that will work wonders to relax you and allow you to slowly release the built-up stress that we all have throughout a busy day.

I have always found exercise to be a great stress-reliever. Try some form of exercise each day, if only for a short time. I love to walk in my neighborhood and enjoy the unique beauty of each season of the year. It doesn't matter what exercise you choose, but it is important to choose some form of exercise that is right and comfortable for you and do it regularly.

Lastly, take time for yourself each day to do some *spiritual* repair to your body and soul. I don't want you to think I am endorsing any particular religion or recommending any particular kind of belief, but I do feel it is important to have a strong belief in a higher power or in a religious faith. At least it is for me. I believe if you are focused outward, rather than inward, if your life is centered more around giving than taking, then better things happen to you physically and mentally.

I am a very spiritual person and I do believe in spiritual healing. The spiritual healing I'm talking about involves one's ability
to find inner peace, be it through some form of meditation, contemplation, prayer, or visualization. Find a place completely to
yourself and just sit quietly and think. Visualize yourself as
happy, healthy, and relaxed. Always the optimist, I visualize
myself as a very statuesque grandmother attending the wedding
of a grandchild, and everyone is saying, "My, doesn't she look
marvelous." For after all, a good positive attitude, a strong dose
of faith, and great expectations are keys to a happy, healthy life.
It worked for my Aunt Rose, and it works for me.

Hormone Replacement Therapy

This is another issue of great controversy today. Before you can
take a stand or ask your doctor where he stands, you need to
know a little bit about hormone replacement therapy and what
it could mean to your health.

The normal female menstrual cycle in premenopausal
women involves the secretion of estrogens followed by progestins from the ovaries. This is followed by a building up and
then shedding of the inner layer of the uterus, causing us to
experience our monthly periods. As we enter menopause, our
body stops producing these estrogens, a fact of life that comes
naturally with the aging process. Along with menopause might
come several unpleasant side effects such as hot flashes, irri-
tability, and depression. Osteoporosis (the loss of calcium in the
bones) is another common problem of women in or past
menopause, causing a variety of problems including weak
bones, painful fractures (particularly to the leg and hip), and
loss of height. Following menopause, a woman's risk for heart
disease also increases.

Replacing the lost estrogens (estrogen replacement therapy, or ERT) can alleviate some or all of these problems. Some experts believe ERT is also effective in reducing the risk of cardiovascular disease. The controversy is this: While no one doubts ERT's potential value to women suffering from severe menopausal symptoms, many physicians feel it increases the risk of both breast cancer and cancer of the uterus (endometrial cancer). The latest scientific studies indicate that low doses of estrogen replacement treatment might be associated with a small increased risk of breast cancer. Estrogen replacement treatment by itself is also associated with a substantially increased risk of cancer of the uterus. As a means of rectifying the problem, adding a second group of hormones, progestins, to the therapy has been recommended. Studies indicate that by adding these low-dose progestins the risk of endometrial cancer is greatly reduced. But what about the risk of breast cancer? This is where the studies are most controversial. In the opinion of some experts, the adding of low-dose progestins to low-dose estrogens actually increases the risk of breast cancer. Other medical authorities disagree, saying that the studies do not indicate a heightened risk of breast cancer to women on estrogen replacement therapy in the vast majority of situations. They say that if there are breast cancer cells somewhere in your body that will ultimately show up as a recurrence, hormone replacement might affect the growth of those cells (either by speeding them up or slowing them down). These experts feel that receiving hormone replacement therapy is an informed-decision issue.

Clearly, there is still much to be learned in this area. Most experts will agree, however, that a woman with a personal history of breast cancer should be disease-free for at least five years before considering hormone replacement therapy for herself. Any woman considering this treatment option should discuss it thoroughly with her gynecologist. A former breast cancer patient should discuss it with her oncologist as well.

In 1992, The National Cancer Institute began sponsorship of the Breast Cancer Prevention Trial, a large study that will enroll sixteen thousand women in the United States and Canada. The trial is using the anti-estrogen drug tamoxifen to test whether it will prevent breast cancer in women who have never had breast cancer. All women ages thirty-five to fifty-nine are eligible if they are at increased risk for breast cancer. All women age sixty and older are eligible if they have not had breast cancer. Participants take tamoxifen or a placebo daily for five years. Women participating in the study might experience some annoying side effects such as hot flashes, nausea, vaginal discharge, or vaginal dryness. Every effort is made to minimize these symptoms. The drug might also lower the risk of heart disease and osteoporosis. Results should be available in five to seven years.

Data tracking women *with* breast cancer who have taken tamoxifen for two to five years is very encouraging. The data suggests a 40- to 50-percent lower incidence of a second breast cancer in the group taking tamoxifen, as compared to the group taking a placebo. Tracking of this group has gone beyond the five-year period during which tamoxifen was taken, in some cases as long as twelve years. Note: As we have discussed earlier, patients taking tamoxifen have a small risk of developing a type of uterine cancer called endometrial cancer. If you are interested in participating in the Breast Cancer Prevention Trial, please contact your physician for his advice or the National Cancer Institute's Cancer Information Service at 1-800 4 CANCER.

CHAPTER TWELVE

Gearing up Again:
If Cancer Recurs

When breast cancer is first diagnosed, most of us experience a plethora of emotions. Fright, anger, confusion, and desperation seem to take over in the beginning as the realization of our own mortality sinks in. As a woman learns more about her options and understands all that can be done to combat the disease, some of those emotions are replaced by hope and an overwhelming feeling of strength and determination. Ideally, she will get through the ordeal and will gain a better appreciation for life while living each new day to the fullest.

When you get into a tight place and everything goes against you till it seems you cannot hold on a minute longer, Never give up, For that is just the place or time That the tide will turn.

HARRIET BEECHER STOWE

It doesn't always happen that way. After bravely enduring one or more types of treatment, even the most noble of fighters can be faced with the devastating news that her cancer has recurred. A recurring cancer is a tumor growth in the area of the original cancer site, either in the remaining breast tissue, the skin, the chest wall, or nearby lymph nodes. It might also be a form of metastasis, cancer that has spread through the blood and/or lymph system to other parts of the body such as the bones, liver, lungs, or brain. It is possible that some of the original cancer cells were not destroyed by the first round of treatment. They might have lain dormant for several months or even years before beginning a regrowth.

Having a breast cancer recurrence is not necessarily a death sentence. Many women go on to live full, healthy, and active lives after one or more cancer recurrences. Still, the emotional energy required to gear up again for more treatment after believing that you have beaten the disease can be staggering. A feeling of bitter disappointment combined with rage and despair can be crippling if you allow it to be. This is the time when you will need every bit of courage and positive energy you can muster. "Know, above all else, that this is not your fault," insists Dr. Jimmie Holland, chief of psychiatric services at Memorial Sloan-Kettering in New York. "Release the guilt. A cancer recurrence is not a personal failure, it is a disease."

The treatment options for breast cancer recurrence are the same as for initial breast cancer. If the initial surgery was less extensive, more surgery might be required. Chemotherapy, radiation therapy, and/or hormone therapy might also be suggested, although the dosages might vary according to your specific needs.

Should you be diagnosed with recurrent or metastatic disease, your medical team of experts as well as your emotional support system will need to come up with a new strategy and a new plan of action. Try to find strength in the fact that by now you are a much more knowledgeable and educated cancer patient. Some of the mystery and uncertainty about what to expect from the treatment will be diminished. Knowing what to expect will enable you to better organize your next round of treatment around the rest of your life.

And it is important to go on being as active as possible. Don't give up or give in to this disease. This time you might beat it— once and for all. Remember, others have done it successfully before you. I know many people who have lived sometimes years beyond a medical diagnosis through sheer will and faith. Just stay focused on what you have learned to do to help yourself and stay positive.

If you do not personally know a patient who has survived recurrent or metastatic breast cancer, contact The Susan G. Komen Breast Cancer Foundation, the American Cancer Society, or the National Cancer Institute; these organizations will be able to put you in touch with someone in your area who can give you, firsthand, the hope and courage you need to go on.

CHAPTER THIRTEEN

Joining the
Race for the Cure®

The race for the cure is not the sole responsibility of medical professionals or cancer organizations like the Komen Foundation. The race will not be won until all women take part in it. At this time, there is no cure for breast cancer. But there *is* hope. *If breast cancer is detected in its earliest stages and treated promptly, there is a greater-than-90-percent, five-year survival rate.* When all women are made aware of the seriousness of breast cancer, the importance of early diagnosis, and the various treatment options, thousands more women's lives will be saved.

Nothing was ever accomplished by sitting around on your duff!

ELLIE GOODMAN

In taking the time to read this book, you have taken the first step in preparing yourself and those you love to run the race against breast cancer. Please, go a step further. Join with us: help save lives in your community. Give women what they need most—knowledge. Teach other women what you now know—*mammograms save lives.*

The Susan G. Komen Breast Cancer Foundation, in conjunction with the National Cancer Institute, has formulated a list of ways to successfully spread the word. If you have often wanted to do something for your community but didn't know where to begin, perhaps these suggestions will inspire you. Think how enriched your own life could be if you were partly responsible for helping save even one woman from suffering.

- Volunteer to serve for one of the many Race for the Cure® events across the country or join a Komen chapter. Call The Komen Foundation National Toll-free Breast Care Helpline 1-800 I'M AWARE (1-800-462-9273) to get information about a race or chapter in your area.

- Make a commitment. If you belong to a women's organization, ask it to make a commitment to educating women about early detection, which includes breast self-examination, regular clinical examinations by a health-care professional, and screening mammography. If you don't belong to an organization, call one that interests you and tell the leader of your idea—perhaps the PTA, a working women's group, your bowling league, tennis team, etc.

- Canvas your neighborhood, your child's playgroup, your church or synagogue with educational materials about breast cancr and the importance of mammograms.

- Put information about breast cancer and the importance of screening for breast cancer on the Internet or other computer networks.

- If you are a federal employee, encourage your fellow workers to designate The Susan G. Komen Foundation in your local CFC Campaign.

- Cosponsor a "Women's Health Fair." Work with the local hospital, medical center, or cancer society to put on such an event. Arrange for local healthcare professionals to talk about the importance of mammography and to screen women at a low cost.

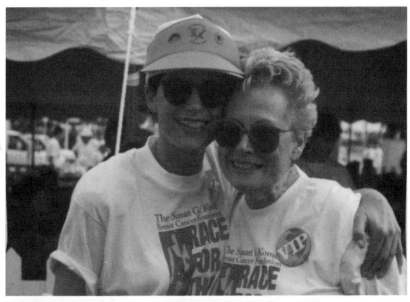

With Mom at the Race for the Cure® in Palm Beach, Florida (1994).

With Zora Brown, founder of the Breast Cancer Resource Committee (1994). *(Photo by Sylvia R. Dunnavant)*

With Norman and my stepdaughter, Brenda Brinker Bottum, recipient of the Gretchen Poston award for her volunteer work with the Baltimore Race for the Cure® (1994).

With Mrs. Tipper Gore, wife of Vice President Al Gore, and Elizabeth A. Hart, 1994 Komen Foundation Chairman (1994).

- Call a local Komen Chapter or Race For the Cure® affiliate to help organize mammography education programs. Work with your employer and with other major employers in your area to sponsor screenings education programs.
- Suggest a women-only brown-bag lunch seminar at your place of employment, where local healthcare professionals can speak on screening mammography, breast self-examination, and clinical breast examinations as early-detection methods.
- Work to extend insurance coverage of mammography. If your health coverage does not include screening mammograms, work with your company's employee insurance coordinator to extend your company's coverage to include this benefit.
- Ask your company's employee insurance coordinator to obtain resource lists from your insurer and make them available to all employees.
- Set up a bulletin board display. Develop a display of posters, brochures, and a list of local accredited mammography facilities for your office, club, beauty salon, lingerie shop, department store, or grocery.
- Encourage the local broadcast media to run public service announcements. Prepared PSAs are available from the national office of The Susan G. Komen Breast Cancer Foundation or the American Cancer Society. Ask your local television stations, cable networks, and radio stations if they will play them.
- Inform the community about mammography facilities and costs. Survey local hospitals and freestanding mammography centers about their hours of availability and costs of services. Let your community know the results by writing a letter to the editor.

- Take a group of friends to get a mammogram. Borrow or rent a van and all go together. Then have lunch, see a movie—anything it takes to make the experience a pleasant one.
- Give the gift of mammography for Mother's Day, birthdays, or "Just Because" days.
- Ask for the gift of mammography from someone you love.
- Lobby your congressmen and senators to increase funding on the state and local level for mammography screening and breast cancer research.

Now you know how I feel about the importance of "action," "knowledge," and "taking charge." Do make an effort—do take a stand. By channeling anger and frustration into action, everyone can help make things better.

CHAPTER FOURTEEN

Susan G. Komen Breast Cancer Foundation's Mission

Over the years I have watched the foundation grow from its tiny beginning to what it is today—the nation's largest private funder of research dedicated solely to breast cancer. We have become a national organization with a network of volunteers working through local chapters and Race for the Cure® events in fifty-nine cities throughout thirty-two states and the District of Columbia and we are still expanding. I marvel at what can be done by first *one* person, then two, then ten, then thousands. Each and every contribution along the way, whether of time, talent, or money, has made a difference in the lives of women. I would like to tell you just how far we have come and what kind of exciting and rewarding work is being done as a result.

The primary mission of The Susan G. Komen Breast Cancer Foundation is *to eradicate breast cancer as a life-threatening disease by advancing research, education, screening, and treatment.* To that end, literally thousands of dedicated volunteers, complemented by a small Foundation staff, work tirelessly year after year to fulfill that mission.

Research

Research holds the key to the cure of this devastating disease, and we are determined to continue to support scientists in this endeavor. We are well within reach of a day when breast cancer will be both preventable and curable. The foundation is funding cutting-edge research that could be the key to unlocking the mystery.

At the publication of this book, the foundation has raised more than $39 million and has funded more than two hundred national research grants using a peer-review selection process approved by the National Cancer Institute. Each year at our National Awards Luncheon in October we honor outstanding achievement in research, voluntarism, community service, and philanthropy. The Komen Award for Scientific Distinction is given for excellence in basic or clinical research. It is important for us to recognize outstanding work in the field of breast cancer research, for in doing so it raises awareness and spurs others to continue the elusive search for a cure.

Only recently have scientists discovered the BRCA-1 gene, which is a breast cancer gene associated with a family history of early-onset breast cancer and ovarian cancer. A Komen National Research Grant recipient was one of the first scientists to conduct genetic research in the field of breast cancer. The researcher is studying genetics within families where multiple female members have breast cancer. The research is fascinating and will hopefully lead to diagnostic testing to determine a woman's risk of familial breast cancer.

We are funding research on Magnetic Resonance Imaging (MRI). This is a new, experimental technique that uses the interaction between magnetism and radio waves to picture the structure of biological tissues. MRI is too costly to replace mammography as a screening procedure, but might be useful as a sophisticated diagnostic tool in cases where conventional methods cannot provide a diagnosis.

I can't begin to tell you of all the fascinating research, both basic and clinical, that we are funding at major institutions across the country. But I can tell you this: We will not stop until a cure is found. My goal, and the goal of the wonderful people with whom I work, is to be out of the business of funding breast cancer research as quickly as possible. What an accomplishment it will be to write the final chapter of this foundation because we have found a cure.

Race for the Cure®

Our Race for the Cure® series, which originated in Dallas in 1983, has been a phenomenal success. It has grown to fifty-seven races in 1995 and is still growing. It has become the largest women's five-kilometer series in the country. Marilyn Tucker Quayle served as our first National Honorary Race Chair, and now Francie Larrieu-Smith, five-time Olympian, serves in that capacity. As well as being a road race for serious runners, this emotionally charged event attracts many first-time and recreational runners. Participants include the young and old, runners and walkers, those participating "in honor" or "in memory" of friends and family members, and especially those wonderful "survivors" wearing neon-pink visors. They are our inspiration and the reason to continue the work we do.

In each race community, 75 percent of the proceeds are used within the local community to fund breast cancer education, screening, and treatment projects. Because of the Race for the Cure®, thousands of women who could not afford mammograms are being screened and are being taught positive breast health practices.

The remaining 25 percent of race proceeds are used to fund national research grants in such areas as genetics, magnetic resonance imaging, hormonal and drug therapies, education, and other promising areas of basic and clinical research. Discoveries are being made almost daily that increase our knowledge of this disease.

The Race for the Cure® is an enormously effective way to reach many, many women with the message that breast cancer is not necessarily fatal if breast self-examination and mammography become routine. It is supported by generous, committed national sponsors, local sponsors, and by the countless volunteers who make it all work. Call the Komen National Toll-free Breast Care Helpline at 1-800 I'M AWARE (1-800-462-9273) to determine if there is a race in your area where you can volunteer.

Education

Until prevention strategies or a cure can be found, early detection is the most cost-effective approach to breast cancer. Through its Affiliate network, The Komen Foundation sponsors educational activities to help women understand the importance of a positive breast health program and help to cope when the disease has been diagnosed.

Being diagnosed with breast cancer can have devastating effects upon the patient, as well as the family and friends. Supporting the needs of the patient and those closest to her is of paramount importance to The Komen Foundation. As a result of work being done throughout the Affiliate network, many programs have evolved that address not only the needs of the breast cancer patient, but the needs of the family as well. There is a growing number of support groups for children and families of breast cancer patients.

The Komen Foundation's National Toll-free Breast Care Helpline, 1-800 I'M AWARE, went on-line in October 1989. It is answered by trained, caring volunteers who provide helpful information and resources to individuals with breast health or breast cancer concerns. For immediate feedback to questions or moral support, patients, their family and friends can call and speak with one of these volunteers, who for the most part are survivors themselves. I receive letters from women across the country expressing their thanks for the kindness shown by our Helpline volunteers.

In addition to our educational efforts year-round, we focus considerable efforts every October during National Breast Cancer Awareness Month to blanket radio, TV, and print media with information, special interest stories, facts, special promotions, public service announcements, and anything else that will educate the public. Every major magazine and newspaper in the country, as well as corporations and organizations that recognize the need and the responsibility, address the issue of breast cancer. Physicians and healthcare facilities across the country offer no-cost or low-cost mammography to qualified candidates on National Mammography Day.

Advocacy

The Komen Foundation has carried out its mission to eradicate breast cancer as a life-threatening disease by raising millions of private funds to advance research, education, screening and treatment throughout the country. While the foundation funds many programs on its own, it has become a leader in forging government links at the federal, state and local level. The foundation matches funds to those supplied by the government to support programs that fight breast cancer. As a result, the foundation has become a private sector partner of the government, and part of the solution in the fight against breast cancer.

Because the foundation actively raises and spends private funds to fight breast cancer, it holds a unique leadership role as an advocate on breast cancer issues. The Komen Foundation has been a leading advocate for insurance reform that offers mandatory coverage of screening mammography, informed legislation and screening vans for the indigent and medically underserved.

Officers and friends of the Komen Foundation have testified in congressional hearings on behalf of breast cancer awareness, increased federal funding for research, and in support of the 1992 Mammography Quality Standards Act. The act requires all screening facilities, equipment and technicians to be accredited by a government approved accrediting body such as the American College of Radiology. Our efforts were key in its passage.

The foundation has long been a leading advocate for increased funding of breast cancer research and started pursuing this goal in 1983, when the federal budget for breast cancer research at the National Cancer Institute was $33 million. Today, at NCI alone, that figure is $313 million. This figure does not include funding at the National Institutes of Health for the National Action Plan on Breast Cancer—on whose steering committee the foundation serves—or at the Department of Defense for the Army Breast Cancer Research Program. Komen actively supported passage by Congress in 1993 of the $210 million "peace dividend" to establish this program at DOD, and the foundation has a seat on the Integration Panel that makes recommendations to the Department of Defense for distribution of research funds. I have been privileged to serve by presidential appointment on the National Cancer Advisory Board and the President's Cancer Panel.

In 1994 and 1995, Komen Chapter and Race for the Cure® affiliates from all parts of the nation went to Washington, D.C. to visit senators and congressmen and discuss with them the key public health and public policy issues surrounding breast cancer.

These are giant steps forward in the fight against breast cancer; but we are continuing our advocacy efforts to increase federal funding of breast cancer research and to make an impact where health care legislation is concerned.

It is important that each and every one of us utilize whatever political networks or political connections we have at the local, regional and national levels. We must flex our political muscle to create a national consciousness about breast cancer. Whatever you can personally do to impact the system, you should do it. Because of my work with The Komen Foundation, I have gained some access to government, and I continue to speak out about critical issues. But each of us needs to be involved in raising the level of awareness of breast cancer issues and raising the national consciousness in terms of solving the problems.

Outreach

One of the primary goals of the Komen Foundation is to focus attention and resources on the critical problem of breast cancer in minority populations and the medically underserved. Special emphasis is placed on developing and funding outreach programs for these groups where the death rate is high due to lack of awareness of good breast health care. Examples of important programs The Komen Foundation has funded are the "Patient

Navigator" program developed at New York's Harlem Hospital and "Witnessing in the Delta," developed in cooperation with the University of Arkansas Cancer Research Center. As Director of the Cancer Control Center of Harlem, Dr. Harold P. Freeman developed "Patient Navigator," a pilot program designed to assist cancer patients and those at high risk to alleviate the institutional barriers to diagnostic and treatment services in a public hospital system.

As I have shared with you in this book, getting through the maze of paperwork, options, decisions, and other problems associated with breast cancer is overwhelming. And I was an educated breast cancer patient! Through this program, trained "Patient Navigators" volunteer to work one-on-one with patients to guide them through all phases of diagnosis and treatment. This pilot program has proven to be a highly effective and efficient system that is being used as a model in other hospitals across the country. We were very proud to award Dr. Freeman the foundation's 1994 Award for Community Service for his work on behalf of breast cancer patients and especially his work on behalf of minorities and the medically underserved.

Recognizing that, in general, participation by minorities and indigent populations in breast cancer screening and education programs is low, and that these groups have resulting higher mortality rates, an intervention program was developed at the University of Arkansas Cancer Research Center to train volunteers to go into rural areas and teach breast health education to African-American women.

The program sought to work through a network of churches in rural communities. Aptly named "Witnessing in the Delta," the program is directed by Dr. Deborah O. Irwin, Ph.D, and her colleague Dr. Thea Spatz at the University of Arkansas Cancer Research Center, and fills a critical need in the Arkansas Delta.

Volunteers "witness" about their triumphs over breast cancer, teach breast self-examination, educate about the importance of early detection, and spread the good news that breast cancer, when detected early, need not be a death sentence. In 1994, Dr. Irwin and three of the Arkansas "witnesses" made a presentation to members of the administration's Domestic Policy staff to highlight the program as a model for other communities and demonstrate how the program could work in a number of other environments.

In April 1994, more than three hundred African-American and Hispanic women convened for the first Minority Breast Cancer Awareness Day in Washington, D.C. We were proud to be a part of the sponsorship of this event, which brought together congressional black and Hispanic caucus members, celebrities from across the country, and breast cancer advocacy groups, all of whom were challenged to become more active in their communities as intermediaries in the battle against breast cancer. It is our hope to strengthen this outreach and make a difference in the mortality rate among minorities and the medically underserved.

In cooperation with the Center for Disease Control (CDC), The Komen Foundation is developing a model breast health outreach program for Hispanic women over the age of fifty. This program will coordinate its educational outreach with existing state and local programs and increase the number of Hispanic women over fifty participating in breast and cervical screening programs. Special materials will be produced in Spanish and the program will be staffed by trained volunteers.

As you can see, we are working on many, many fronts to battle this disease, and we promise to continue that work for as long as it takes. If this book has helped you, please share it with someone else.

The Komen Foundation is battling a formidable enemy, one that's gaining momentum. We're not fighting for principal, or some obscure cause.

We're Fighting for Our Very Lives. And to Win We Need You To Join Our Battle.

Through educating yourself about the disease, sharing your knowledge, taking preventive measures, volunteering to help our battle or contributing...we need you!

Please write or call:
- for breast cancer information
- to receive our newsletter
- to volunteer
- for a list of Komen Chapters or Race Committees
- to contribute to the cause

The Susan G. Komen Breast Cancer Foundation
5005 LBJ Freeway, Suite 370
Dallas, TX 75244
214/450-1777 214/450-1710 (fax)

National Tollfree Breast Care Helpline
1/800 I'M AWARE
(1-800-462-9273)

Komen Affiliate Network

In early 1995, The Susan G. Komen Breast Cancer Foundation had affiliates in fifty-nine cities throughout thirty-two states and the District of Columbia.

Please call our 1-800-I'M AWARE Helpline to learn how you can join in the activites in a city near you.

Birmingham, Alabama
Phoenix, Arizona
Little Rock, Arkansas
Orange County, California
Sacramento, California
San Diego, California
San Francisco, California
Aspen, Colorado
Colorado Springs, Colorado
Denver, Colorado
New Britain, Connecticut
Washington, D.C.
Jacksonville, Florida
West Palm Beach, Florida
Atlanta, Georgia
Honolulu, Hawaii
Chicago, Illinois
Decatur, Illinois
Peoria, Illinois
Indianapolis, Indiana
Davenport, Iowa
Des Moines, Iowa
Wichita, Kansas
Monroe, Louisiana
New Orleans, Louisiana
Shreveport, Louisiana
Baltimore, Maryland
Boston, Massachusetts
Detroit, Michigan
Minneapolis, Minnesota

Kansas City, Missouri
Helena, Montana
Omaha, Nebraska
Albany, New York
Syracuse, New York
New York, New York
Princeton, New Jersey
Cleveland, Ohio
Columbus, Ohio
Toledo, Ohio
Oklahoma City, Oklahoma
Portland,Oregon
Philadelphia, Pennsylvania
Pittsburgh, Pennsylvania
Scranton, Pennsylvania
Charleston, South Carolina
Greenville, South Carolina
Memphis, Tennessee
Nashville, Tennessee
Amarillo, Texas
Austin, Texas
Dallas, Texas
El Paso, Texas
Ft. Worth, Texas
Houston, Texas
Lubbock, Texas
Plano, Texas
Manchester, Vermont
Seattle, Washington

CHAPTER FIFTEEN

And Now…

Now, a number of years after my original diagnosis, there is still a little panic that wells up inside me whenever it is time for a checkup. But I take a deep breath, say a little prayer, and go anyway. I do everything I know to keep healthy, and I really work hard at it. Still, I try not to forget to look up now and then and say, "Thanks."

> *To love what you do and feel that it matters—how could anything be more fun?*
>
> KATHARINE GRAHAM

Norman, Eric, and I continue to cherish our life together. But in January 1993, I was not sure where that life was going. Norman suffered a serious head injury in a polo accident and was in a coma for three weeks. You can imagine the old memories that flooded back into my mind as I sat by his hospital bed, wondering if this man who had brought so much joy into my life was now to be taken away from me. It was a situation I could not conceive nor endure.

Summoning strength I never knew I had, I stayed with Norman constantly. I talked to him and read to him day and night, when I was not sure he could even hear me. I was not going to lose this man if I could help it. Norman always stayed physically fit, so he had that in his favor. He is also a fighter, just like I am, and I was determined that together, with family, friends, and the best medical team we could assemble, we would pull him through this ordeal, too. And I'm happy to tell you we did. It has taken months of rehabilitation, but with incredible courage and strength, Norman has fought back. He has returned to the helm of his company and is doing very well.

I do not know why this happened to us, I only know I am extremely thankful and grateful that Norman's life was spared. Maybe Suzy's legacy to me was what she taught me about hope and prayer and positive thinking. Living every day to its fullest now seems so much more important to us and brings into sharper focus the real importance of family and friends.

Eric is in college now and is, as always, the joy of my life. My parents, niece, nephew, and brother-in-law have rebuilt their lives, but live constantly with the void of Suzy's absence.

My work at The Komen Foundation continues, though I have turned over the day-to-day management to a wonderful group of volunteers and staff. As I have told you, we are still raising money and awareness. It is especially gratifying to me to see the problem of breast cancer slowly but surely making its way into the limelight. A few years ago, no one would talk about this disease. It is such an enormous contrast to the days when we began The Komen Foundation and so many people blushed at the mere mention of the words "breasts." Doors were slammed in our faces over and over again when we were asking people to contribute and become a part of this important activity. Fear was so enormously prevailing, from the bedroom to the boardroom. Today it is freely spoken about in every circle. This new awareness and acceptance is largely due to the generosity of some of the country's most well-known celebrities and public policy leaders who have been willing to speak out on the cause, and leaders of corporate America willing to commit precious dollars to help find a cure. It has now become fashionable to be informed about breast cancer.

I would like to see more of it. I would like to see still more funds being set aside nationally for breast cancer research and education. Since the Pap Smear has been accepted as part of a woman's routine health check, the mortality rate for cervical cancer has decreased by 75 percent. I know the same could happen for breast cancer if women considered a screening mammogram part of a routine examination. I believe that if the entire medical community—including physicians, nurses, and patients—were to think in terms of preventive medicine rather than just curative medicine, more lives would be saved.

Although it is clear we are each born with a genetic composition that is sometimes beyond our control, I have to believe that practicing good preventive health care, maintaining a good diet, getting at least moderate exercise, and creating a good, spiritual, stress-controlled environment would really lead to better outcomes for all of us. Most people still only go to the doctor when they feel "sick." How nice it would be if we could partner with our physicians and develop a "living plan" that would help keep us from being ill and help ensure a longer, healthier life.

I have now spent nearly two decades involved in this cause, from the time my sister was diagnosed, to the present day. Breast cancer has virtually become my "career" over the years, and I want to continue my work to create more opportunities to fund the work we do.

I am very proud of the work The Komen Foundation has done and proud of the public policy work I have been able to do for the government. Serving for eight years under Presidents Reagan and Bush on the National Cancer Advisory Board has been a distinct privilege, as I was one of only six laypersons appointed. In 1991, President Bush appointed me to the three-member President's Cancer Panel where I chaired a special sub-committee on breast cancer. This extremely rewarding work has strengthened my commitment and made me realize just how much more work there is to be done.

Because of the years of work in this field, I now serve on the boards of two publicly-held healthcare companies and am an active public speaker. Many honors have been bestowed upon me for "courage" and "hard work" and other altruistic motives, but the promise made so many years ago to Suzy is still why I keep going and continues to drive everything I do.

It is sad to say, but since I first published this book in 1990, one hundred eighty-two thousand women each year have been diagnosed with breast cancer (one every three minutes)—and forty-six thousand have died each year. Tragically, those are people you cherished and people I cherished—and miss terribly. But on the positive side, I know the work being done in educating women about early detection is saving lives. *I know it.*

Ten years from now, when I see a significant improvement in the mortality rate, better preventative measures, and I hope a cure for breast cancer—and I feel certain that I will—I will know that my sister is resting in peace because her final wishes have been fulfilled. We are winning. The victors are our mothers, our sisters, our daughters, our friends...ourselves.

A Breast Cancer Glossary

There are some terms you will see over and over again within this book and hear often in your doctor's office. I have tried to explain each term as it came up in the text, but I know from experience that "cancer talk" can sound like a foreign language at first. And foreign languages are easy to forget. The Susan G. Komen Breast Cancer Foundation has put together a quick reference list of common terms to refresh your memory at a glance. The definitions are short and uncomplicated, meant only to give you a fast, easy idea of what a word means. For more detailed information, use the index to find the term within the text, or ask your doctor.

Adjuvant Therapy: cancer treatment such as radiation or chemotherapy used in addition to the primary form of treatment, which is generally surgery.

Alopecia: hair loss. Often occurs as a result of chemotherapy.

Anesthesia: entire or partial loss of feeling or sensation produced by drugs or gases.

Antiemetic: a medicine to prevent or relieve nausea and vomiting.

Areola: the circular field of dark-colored skin surrounding the nipple.

Aspiration: withdrawal of fluid from a cyst with a hypodermic needle.

Axilla: the underarm area.

Benign: noncancerous (usually not life-threatening).

Biopsy: removal of suspicious tissue for examination under a microscope for diagnosis.

Core Needle Biopsy: removal of a cylinder of tissue with a large diameter needle from a growth or mass for microscopic diagnosis. Sometimes referred to as stereotactic biopsy.

Excisional Biopsy: removal of an entire growth for diagnosis.

Fine Needle Aspiration Biopsy: removal of cells with a small diameter needle, from a growth or mass for microscopic diagnosis.

Incisional Biopsy: surgical removal of a portion of a growth or mass for microscopic diagnosis.

Bone Scan: a picture of all the bones in the body taken two hours after injection of a radioactive tracer.

Bone (skeletal) Survey: X rays of the entire skeleton.

Breast Cancer: an uncontrolled growth of abnormal breast cells.

Breast Implant: an "envelope" containing silicone or saline (or both) used to restore breast form.

Breast Self-Exam: a method used by women to become familiar with the normal appearance and feel of their breast tissue so that if a change occurs, it will be detected early.

CAT Scan: a cross-sectional view of the entire body through X ray, which might show cancer or metastases earlier and more accurately than other imaging methods.

Chemotherapy: treatment with drugs to destroy cancer cells; often used to supplement surgery and/or radiation or to treat recurrent cancer.

Cyst: a fluid-filled sac or cavity, usually harmless, which can be removed by aspiration. See "aspiration."

Cytotoxic: cell-killing.

Duct Ectasia: see "mammary duct ectasia."

Ductal Papillomas: noncancerous breast tumor, arising in the breast duct, usually cannot be felt. Commonly found in women forty-five to fifty. Generally appears as either a bloody or clear nipple discharge.

Endocrine Manipulation: treating breast cancer by changing the hormonal balance of the body instead of using cell-killing drugs (chemotherapy).

Estrogen: a female hormone important to reproduction, which is produced by the ovaries and the adrenal glands and might be needed by some cancers for growth. See "hormones."

Estrogen Receptor Assay (ERA): a laboratory test performed on a malignant breast tumor to determine if the tumor needs estrogen to grow.

Fat Necrosis: destruction of fat cells due to trauma or injury that can cause a noncancerous lump.

Fibroadenoma: a noncancerous, solid breast tumor most commonly found in younger women.

Fibrocystic Breast Condition: a noncancerous breast condition sometimes resulting in painful cysts or lumpy breasts. It can be accompanied by discomfort or pain that fluctuates with menstrual cycle.

Flow Cytometry: a test done on cancerous tissue to determine the growth rate of malignant cells and the presence of abnormal chromosomes. Indicates aggressiveness of tumor.

Frozen Section: a technique in which a part of the biopsy tissue is frozen immediately and a thin slice is then mounted on a microscope slide, enabling a pathologist to analyze it in just a few minutes for a diagnosis.

Halsted (Radical) Mastectomy: see "mastectomy."

Hormone Therapy: see "endocrine manipulation."

Hormones: substances made by the body that regulate the activity of certain cells or organs. They are largely responsible for reproductive function and aspects of appearance that distinguish the sexes.

Hormone Receptor Assay: a diagnostic test to determine whether a breast cancer's growth is influenced by hormones and can be treated with hormone therapy.

Hysterectomy: surgical removal of the uterus.

Immunotherapy: treatment of cancer by stimulating the body's immune defense system.

Infiltrating Duct Cell Cancer: a cancer that begins in the mammary ducts and spreads to surrounding tissue.

Intravenous (IV): entering the body by way of a vein.

Inverted Nipple: the turning inward of the nipple. Usually a congenital condition, but if it occurs where it has not previously existed, it can be a sign of breast cancer.

Latissimus Dorsi Flap Reconstruction: the latissimus dorsi, a large, flat muscle on the patient's back, along with the overlying skin, is used to reconstruct a breast mound at the mastectomy site. The patient might require an expander or implant if there is not enough tissue to achieve an appropriate volume.

Linear Accelerator: a machine that produces high-energy X rays or electrons to treat cancer.

Liver Scan: a way of visualizing the liver by injecting into the bloodstream a radioactive substance which lights up the organ during X ray.

Lump: any kind of mass in the breast (or elsewhere in the body).

Lumpy Breasts: see "fibrocystic breast condition."

Lumpectomy: a surgical procedure in which only the cancerous tumor and a ring of surrounding normal breast tissue are removed, leaving the remaining normal breast tissue intact.

Usually some of the underarm lymph nodes are removed with another incision. This procedure is followed by radiation.

Lymph Nodes: bean-shaped filtering devices scattered along the vessels of the lymphatic system, which remove wastes and fluids from the body tissues and carry fluids that help the body fight infection. Those found in the underarm (axilla) are most likely to be invaded by breast cancer cells and therefore some are removed during breast cancer surgery.

Lymphedema: swelling in the arm caused by excess fluid that might occur after lymph nodes and vessels have been removed during surgery or following radiation therapy.

Magnetic Resonance Imaging (MRI): a magnet scan; a form of X ray using magnets instead of radiation. MRI gives a more clearly defined picture of fatty tissue than X ray.

Malignant: cancerous.

Mammary Duct Ectasia: a noncancerous breast condition resulting from the inflammation and enlargement of the ducts behind the nipple. Generally, women are asymptomatic; however, mammographic calcifications might indicate its presence. No treatment is necessary if the woman is not experiencing any symptoms (burning, pain, or itching of the nipple area).

Mammary Glands: the breast glands that produce and carry milk, by way of the mammary ducts, to the nipples during pregnancy and breast-feeding.

Mammography/Mammogram: an X ray of the breast for screening and diagnosis of breast cancer.

A screening mammogram is an X ray taken in an asymptomatic (no symptoms) woman to detect any abnormality that might indicate early signs of breast cancer.

A diagnostic mammogram is an X ray taken to further evaluate an already palpable lump or some other abnormality or an abnormal screening mammogram.

A baseline mammogram is an initial screening mammogram to establish a basis for comparison to subsequent mammograms.

Mastectomy: surgical removal of the breast and some surrounding tissue.

Modified Radical Mastectomy: the most common type of mastectomy performed today. The breast, breast skin, nipple, areola, and underarm lymph nodes are removed, while the chest muscles are saved.

Prophylactic Mastectomy: a procedure sometimes recommended for patients at very high risk for developing cancer in one or both breasts.

Subcutaneous mastectomy: done before cancer is detected, removes the breast tissue but leaves the outer skin, areola, and nipple intact. (This is not a suitable cancer operation.)

Radical Mastectomy (Halsted Radical): the surgical removal of the breast, breast skin, nipple, areola, chest muscles, and underarm lymph nodes. Rarely done today.

Segmental Mastectomy (Partial Mastectomy): a surgical procedure in which only a portion of the breast is removed, including the cancer and a surrounding margin of healthy breast tissue. See also "lumpectomy."

Medical Oncologist: a physician who specializes in the treatment of cancer using chemotherapy or hormone therapy.

Menopause: the time in a woman's life when the menstrual cycle ends and the ovaries produce lower levels of hormones. Usually occurs between the ages of forty-five and fifty-five.

Metastasis: the spread of cancer from one part of the body to another through the lymphatic system or the bloodstream. The cells in the new cancer location are the same type as those in the original site.

Microsurgery: the suturing and reattachment of blood vessels under the magnification of the operating microscope.

Oncogenes: growth-regulating genes that can cause tumors when activated.

One-Step Procedure: a procedure in which a surgical biopsy is performed under general anesthesia and, if cancer is found, a mastectomy or lumpectomy is done immediately, as part of the same operation. It should be noted that this is no longer the standard procedure unless the patient is informed and consents in advance to a one-step procedure.

Oophorectomy: surgical removal of the ovaries.

Palliative Therapy: a treatment that might relieve symptoms without curing the disease.

Partial Mastectomy: see "mastectomy."

Pathologist: a physician with special training in diagnosing diseases from samples of tissues.

Palpation: examining with the hands to check for changes or abnormalities.

Permanent Section: a technique in which thin slices of biopsy tissue are mounted on a slide to be examined under a microscope by a pathologist in order to establish a diagnosis. Usually takes three working days to receive the final pathology report.

Progesterone Receptor Assay (PRA): a test that must be done on cancerous tissue to see if a breast cancer is hormone-dependent and can be treated by hormone therapy. Used as a check on the results of the "estrogen receptor assay."

Prosthesis, Breast: an artificial form that can be worn underneath clothing after a mastectomy.

Radiation Therapy: treatment with high-energy X rays to destroy cancer cells.

Radiation Oncologist: a physician specifically trained in the use of high-energy X rays to treat cancer.

Radiologist: a physician who specializes in diagnosis of diseases by the use of X rays.

Reconstruction: a way to recreate the breast's shape after a natural breast has been removed; various surgical procedures are available. Sometimes performed immediately (at the time of mastectomy) or delayed several months or years.

Recurrence: reappearance of cancer at the same site (local), near the site (regional), or in other areas of the body (metastatic or distant).

Silicone Gel: medical-grade silicone rubber in gel form (similar to consistency of the normal breast) used in implants. Available only through clinical trials.

Staging: certain tests and examinations done before any type of definitive treatment to determine if the cancer has spread.

Transverse Rectus Abdominus Myocutaneous Flap (TRAM): To create a chest muscle and breast mound, the surgeon transfers one of the two abdominal muscles, technically called Transverse Rectus Abdominus Myocutaneous, from the stomach to the chest. This procedure is commonly called a "TRAM." This flap of muscle, skin, and fat is shaped into the contour of the opposite breast. If there is enough abdominal tissue available, no implant is needed. This procedure also tightens the abdominal muscles, giving rise to the term "tummy tuck" procedure. The patient will have a scar across the lower abdomen in addition to the mastectomy scar on her chest. Because there are, in effect, two surgeries being performed, recovery might be prolonged.

Tumor: an abnormal growth or mass of tissue; can be either cancerous or noncancerous.

Two-Step Procedure: when surgical biopsy and further surgical treatment are performed at two separate times. Compare to "one-step procedure."

Ultrasonography/Ultrasound—Breast: a noninvasive procedure (a procedure that does not require cutting into the skin) using a sound wave imaging technique to examine the breast. Ultrasound might be helpful in distinguishing between solid masses and cysts. Unlike mammography, ultrasound cannot detect microcalcifications that might be present in the breast, nor does it identify small tumors.

X rays: electromagnetic radiations which can, at low levels, produce images that can diagnose cancer and, at high levels, destroy cancer cells.

Resource Guide

AMC Cancer Research Center
  Cancer Information and Counseling Line
  Cancer Intervention Division
  1600 Pierce Street
  Denver, Colorado 80214
  1-800-525-3777
Dedicated to cancer prevention and control research and meeting cancer survivors' information and counseling needs. Hotline provides information on symptoms, diagnosis, treatment, psycho social issues, support groups, and other valuable resources such as financial aid and transportation services.

American Cancer Society (ACS) and
"Reach to Recovery" Program
  1599 Clifton Road, NE
  Atlanta, Georgia 30329
  1-800-ACS-2345
National tollfree hotline providing information on all forms of cancer and locations for ACS-sponsored "Reach to Recovery" programs.

American College of Radiology
Mammography Accreditation Department
1891 Preston White Drive
Reston, Virginia 22091
1-800-227-6440
Provides lists of facilities with accredited mammography units.

American Medical Association
515 North State Street
Chicago, Illinois 60610
1-312-464-5000

American Society of Clinical Oncology
435 North Michigan Avenue, Suite 1717
Chicago, Illinois 60611
1-312-644-0828

American Society of Plastic and Reconstructive Surgeons
444 East Algonquin Road
Arlington Heights, Illinois 60005
1-800-635-0635 (referral message tape)
An information and referral service for individuals seeking the services of a board-certified plastic surgeon, including those who perform breast reconstruction procedures.

Bosom Buddies
P.O. Box 16687
Phoenix, Arizona 85011-6687
1-602-231-6648 (Hotline)
A nonprofit organization of caring women who have had personal experience dealing with the trauma and challenges of breast cancer. Provides a twenty-four-hour hotline which pairs women with breast cancer with a member of Bosom Buddies.

Sponsors monthly "open-door" meetings and informational newsletter and resource library.

CHEMOcare

231 North Avenue West

Westfield, New Jersey 07090

1-800 55 CHEMO (1-800-552-4366)

National agency that matches a cancer patient with a volunteer cancer survivor who has had a similar cancer experience. Support is provided one-to-one and is free of charge.

Food and Drug Administration's
Breast Implant Information Line

5600 Fishers Lane, Room 16-59

Rockville, Maryland 20857

1-800-532-4440

Provides free comprehensive information packages about breast implants. Call the 800 number twenty-four hours a day and leave your name and address.

"Look Good-Feel Better"

1-800-395-LOOK (1-800-395-5665)

Cosmetics, Toilet and Fragrance Association (CFTA)

Program designed to help women recovering from cancer deal with changes in their appearance resulting from cancer treatment. Print and video material available.

National Alliance of Breast Cancer Organizations (NABCO)

9 East 37th Street—10th Floor

New York, New York 10016

A not-for-profit organization that provides members and health organizations with up-to-date information on all aspects of breast cancer and promotes affordable detection and treatment.

Does not offer diagnosis, treatment, or counseling. Active in efforts to influence policies that pertain directly to breast cancer.

National Breast Cancer Coalition
P.O. Box 66373
Washington D.C. 20035
1-202-296-7477

Advocacy group that educates the public and provides ways for individuals to become involved in the fight to stop the breast cancer epidemic.

National Cancer Institute (NCI)/Cancer Information Service
1-800 4 CANCER (1-800-422-6237)

The Cancer Information Service (CIS) is a nationwide network of nineteen regional offices supported by the National Cancer Institute (NCI), the Federal Government's primary agency for cancer research. Through its toll-free telephone service, the CIS provides accurate, up-to-date information on cancer to patients and their families, health professionals, and the general public. The CIS serves as a resource for state and regional organizations by providing printed materials and technical assistance to cancer education, media campaigns, and community programs. When dialing the 1-800 4 CANCER number your call will automatically be routed to the office that serves the caller's region.

National Coalition for Cancer Survivorship (NCCS)
1010 Wayne Avenue, 5th Floor
Silver Spring, Maryland 20910
1-301-650-8868

NCCS is a network of independent organizations and individuals working in the areas of cancer support and survivorship. The primary goal of the coalition is to generate a nationwide awareness of cancer survivorship. NCCS facilitates communication among people involved with cancer survivorship, promotes the development of cancer support activities, serves as a clearinghouse for information and materials on survivorship, acts as an advocate for survivors of cancer, and encourages study of survivorship.

National Hospice Organization (NHO)

1901 North Moore Street, Suite 901
Arlington, Virginia 22209
1-703-243-5900
Hospice Helpline: 1-800-658-8898

A nonprofit organization and the nation's only advocate for terminally ill patients and their families. Member programs and services include advocacy, educational events and symposia, technical assistance, public relations support, legislative bulletins, and several publications.

National Insurance Consumer Helpline

1-800-942-4242

Trained personnel and licensed agents are available to assist consumers in three important areas. They answer a wide range of questions about various insurance matters, are able to refer consumer complaints to appropriate sources, and send consumer brochures upon request.

National Lymphedema Network

2211 Post Street, Suite 404
San Francisco, California 94115
1-800-541-3259, 415-921-4282 (fax)

A nonprofit organization that disseminates information on the prevention and management of primary and secondary lymphedema to the general public and healthcare professionals, and supports research into the causes, prevention, and management of lymphedema. The NLN offers a quarterly newsletter and a tollfree hotline which provides individuals with emotional support, educational information, referrals to healthcare professionals, treatment centers, local support groups, and exercise programs.

National Surgical Adjuvant Breast and Bowel Project (NSABP)
    230 McKee Place, Suite 402
    Pittsburgh, Pennsylvania 15213
    1-412-383-1400
One of the nation's oldest and largest on going cancer clinical trials.

Physicians Data Query (PDQ)
    Cancer Information Service (CIS)
    1-800 4 CANCER (1-800-422-6237)
A computer database of the NCI that provides cancer information statements, descriptions of research studies, listings of organizations involved in cancer care, and summaries of clinical trials. Includes up-to-date information about screening, supportive care, and treatment. Developed by the National Cancer Institute (NCI). Offers CancerFax, a system that allows users to obtain PDQ information statements by fax machine, and CancerNet, a system that allows users to obtain information through electronic mail.

The Susan G. Komen Breast Cancer Foundation
    5005 LBJ Freeway, Suite 370
    Dallas, Texas 75244
    214-450-1777
    1-800 I'M AWARE (1-800-462-9273)
A national volunteer-based nonprofit organization raising funds to provide educational programs, mammography screening,

and treatment for medically underserved women. As the nation's largest private funder of research dedicated solely to breast cancer, the foundation awards annual grants and fellowships in basic and clinical research. Works in the legislative arena to increase federal funds for breast cancer research and screening. National Tollfree Breast Care Helpline staffed by trained volunteers offers information and resources to individuals with breast health or breast cancer concerns Also provides the names of accredited mammography screening facilities across the country.

Y-Me

212 W. Van Buren, 4th Floor

Chicago, Illinois 60607

1-800-221-2141 9 A.M. to 5 P.M. Central time

312-986-8228 (twenty-four-hour number)

A not-for-profit organization that provides information, hotline counseling, educational programs, and self-help meetings for breast cancer patients, their families, and friends. Provides information on public policy and legislative activities related to breast cancer. Offers workshops for health professionals, technical assistance, a resource library, and newsletter. Y-Me maintains a prosthesis and wig bank for women with financial need. If appropriate size is available, Y-Me will mail a wig and/or breast prosthesis anywhere in the country. A nominal handling fee is requested.

YWCA of the USA Encore Plus Program

624 9th Street NW, 3rd Floor

Washington, D.C. 20001

A system of health promotion through education, clinical service delivery, and patient "navigation" and advocacy. Community-based program targeting women over fifty in need of early detection education, breast and cervical cancer screening, and support services. Also provides women under treatment and recovering from breast cancer a unique, combined peer group support and exercise program.

Index